Be
Incredibly
Sexy

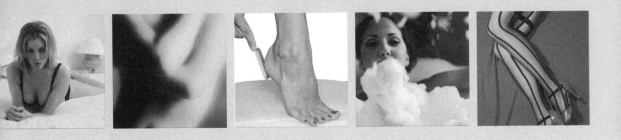

52 Brilliant Ideas
one good idea can change your life

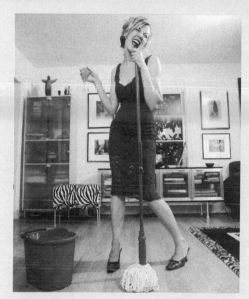

Be Incredibly Sexy

A Crash Course in Getting Your Groove On—and Keeping It There

Helena Frith Powell

A Perigee Book

A PERIGEE BOOK
Published by the Penguin Group
Penguin Group (USA) Inc.
375 Hudson Street, New York, New York 10014, USA
Penguin Group (Canada), 90 Eglinton Avenue East, Suite 700, Toronto, Ontario M4P 2Y3, Canada
(a division of Pearson Penguin Canada Inc.)
Penguin Books Ltd., 80 Strand, London WC2R 0RL, England
Penguin Group Ireland, 25 St. Stephen's Green, Dublin 2, Ireland (a division of Penguin Books Ltd.)
Penguin Group (Australia), 250 Camberwell Road, Camberwell, Victoria 3124, Australia
(a division of Pearson Australia Group Pty. Ltd.)
Penguin Books India Pvt. Ltd., 11 Community Centre, Panchsheel Park, New Delhi—110 017, India
Penguin Group (NZ), 67 Apollo Drive, Rosedale, North Shore 0745, Auckland, New Zealand
(a division of Pearson New Zealand Ltd.)
Penguin Books (South Africa) (Pty.) Ltd., 24 Sturdee Avenue, Rosebank, Johannesburg 2196,
South Africa

Penguin Books Ltd., Registered Offices: 80 Strand, London WC2R 0RL, England

While the author has made every efffort to provide accurate telephone numbers and Internet addresses at the time of publication, neither the publisher nor the author assumes any responsibility for errors, or for changes that occur after publication. Further, the publisher does not have any control over and does not assume any responsibility for author or third-party websites or their content.

BE INCREDIBLY SEXY

First American edition: June 2007
Originally published in Great Britain in 2006 by The Infinite Ideas Company Limited.

Perigee trade paperback ISBN: 978-0-399-53344-0

PRINTED IN THE UNITED STATES OF AMERICA

10 9 8 7 6 5 4 3 2 1

Most Perigee Books are available at special quantity discounts for bulk purchases for sales promotions, permiums, fund-raising, or educational use. Special books, or book excerpts, can also be created to fit specific needs. For details, write: Special Markets, Penguin Group (USA) Inc., 375 Hudson Street, New York, New York 10014.

Brilliant ideas

Brilliant features

Each chapter of this book is designed to provide you with an inspirational idea that you can read quickly and put into practice right away.

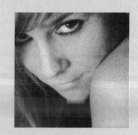

Throughout, you'll find four features that will help you to get right to the heart of the idea:

- *Here's an idea for you* Take it on board and give it a try—right here, right now. Get an idea of how well you're doing so far.

- *Try another idea* If this idea looks like a life-changer, then there's no time to lose. *Try another idea* will point you straight to a related tip to enhance and expand on the first.

- *Defining idea* Words of wisdom from masters and mistresses of the art, plus some interesting hangers-on.

- *How did it go?* If at first you do succeed, try to hide your amazement. If, on the other hand, you don't, then this is where you'll find a Q and A that highlights common problems and how to get over them.

Introduction

Why would you want to buy a book telling you how to be incredibly sexy? You're already incredibly sexy, aren't you? Of course, but just as a golfer is always working on his swing, you should keep working on being sexy.

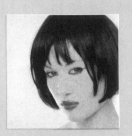

So what is it? What defines sex appeal? And why do some have it when others don't? Defining sex appeal is difficult. Sexual attraction is a mystery and luckily we don't all have the same opinion of what makes someone sexy. Some women find George Clooney irresistible, others prefer John Cleese. Marilyn Monroe is universally regarded as one of the most potent sex symbols ever, but there are men that find her too buxom.

Inès de la Fressange was the original supermodel and one of the most attractive women of her generation. When I asked her what makes somebody sexy her answer was varied. First she said it was important to have the fundamentals, like good teeth: "If a woman is perfectly made up and looks glorious and then smiles to reveal yellow stained teeth, she's not going to be sexy," she says. "Being sexy can also be a movement of the neck or the way your hair falls. It's about small details, the way a woman acts with her hands in her hair. It also has a lot to do with attitude: being happy is sexy, someone who is anguished is not." A friend of mine defines a sexy man as "someone who has a certain something, a certain promise in his smile." So how do you achieve this certain something?

Try to think about what it is that you find sexy in other people, be they film stars or people you come across daily. Is it something in their manner? Is it the way they look? Their voice, their accent, their clothes? One of the quickest ways to become sexy is to look and learn from others. But you have to pick your company carefully. If you play tennis with players that are better than you, you raise your game. If you hang out with sexy, attractive people, you have more of a chance of becoming one as well.

In this book I have tried to point you in the right direction when it comes to discovering your sexier side and also developing areas that can be worked on. For example, you might not immediately think that smell has a huge effect on your sex appeal, but it does. I know a man who claims he fell in love with his wife because she smelled so good. As you will see in Idea 2, smell goes all the way back to the biological basis of sexual attraction and is incredibly important. Some women may not think being pregnant and sexy is possible, but they're so wrong. Pregnancy is one of the sexiest states; your senses are heightened and your body is voluptuous—take advantage of it. You might think you know how to keep your sex life spicy, but do you really?

I cover the fundamentals as well as the details in this book. One goes with the other: you can't be incredibly sexy if you don't have your personal hygiene organized, as well as your intellectually stimulating conversation. There is no point saying something incredibly interesting if your breath makes the person you're talking to want to faint.

But along with more superficial ways you can increase your sex appeal, such as taking better care of your appearance, I think more fundamental issues, like learning to play a musical instrument, are important. Being incredibly sexy is not just about having the right body and underwear. You need to be a sexy person through and through, and that means interesting and fun, with an attractive personality. Someone who does nothing with their life and has no interests is not sexy. My father always said, "If I had a dollar for every woman who told me what an attractive man Onassis is I'd be as rich as he is." Let's face it, the man looked like a toad, but he was rich and powerful. Which made him so interesting he managed to attract two of the greatest female icons of the twentieth century: Maria Callas and Jackie Kennedy.

We can't all look like film stars or opera divas but I hope this book will at least give you the confidence to behave like one, and an incredibly sexy one at that. Remember, having sex is only one good reason for being incredibly sexy. Being sexy gives you confidence, which in turn makes you come across as younger and more dynamic. Being sexy makes you attractive to people and attractive people are often successful people. So, being sexy is about laying a foundation for success. Finally, being sexy means you get to sleep with lots of other sexy people (if you want); a major advantage, but by no means the be all and end all.

1

The confidence factor

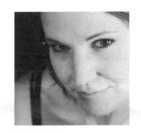

The trick to being sexy is to be confident. You need to believe in and accept yourself. There are, of course, parts of you that you don't like, but don't dwell on them. Exaggerate your good points and work on the bad ones.

When you walk into a room imagine you are Jennifer Lopez or Brad Pitt; don't think "God, I look like a drowned rat and no one will find me attractive."

Sex appeal is not just skin deep, it's also a question of attitude. Confidence is fundamental to sexiness and some people ooze it. They are magnetic, captivating, and not necessarily drop-dead gorgeous. These are usually people who are open, gregarious, amusing, and positive. All attributes that require confidence.

There are days when you will feel like you rule the world and days when you wonder why on earth anyone ever speaks to you. When you have days like the latter, try to think of them as bad hair days. Everyone has them, but they don't last forever. Think to yourself: *There are lots of good things about me.* You could even make a list of all your achievements, such as owning your home, holding down a job, an

Here's an idea for you...

Write down the five things that most attract you to someone. And then figure out how you can adapt them to work for you. For example, someone might have a very sexy tone of voice that you could imitate or maybe a way of sitting that is attractive. Practice small things like this and you'll feel sexier and more confident already.

address book full of friends, a contented cat. Don't forget your best physical attributes. Noting them yourself appears to flag them to other people almost by magic. Soon you'll be receiving compliments.

Set yourself small, achievable goals every week and use them to boost your self-esteem and confidence. Or you could read self-help books. You've made a start by reading this idea so think of some other area of your life you can improve to make you sexier and then get thee to a bookshop (or try out some more Brilliant Ideas).

Try to look at yourself like a stock. Your share price will go up or down, depending on market perception. If things are going well, and you're on a high, your stock will soar; everyone wants to know you. If you're at a low, then your price will drop. And you won't help this drop in price by moping around refusing to go out. You need to work at it until your share price is right up there again. A new haircut, a new outfit, a new career move, anything that will boost you over the bad period. So here are my top five tips for becoming more confident or feigning confidence:

Defining idea...

"All you need in this life are ignorance and confidence; then success is sure."
MARK TWAIN

1. Think about your good points and accentuate them. If you have lovely eyes, say, use them when you're talking to people or flirting.

2. Similarly, DO NOT think about your bad points. You may think the pimple on your chin is the most dramatically dreadful thing to happen to you all year but chances are no one has even noticed it.

3. Feel good, look good. Be healthy. Eat well and exercise. If you feel like you're in shape, you will ooze confidence.

4. A new outfit/haircut/lip gloss can do wonders for your confidence levels. Treat yourself before an important date.

5. It's not about what you've got but what people think you've got. So if you feel your chest is a tad too flat, invest in a Wonderbra. If your lips are not plump enough, then use some lip-liner to accentuate them.

Another good trick is to remain slightly mysterious. If you're confident enough, don't let it all hang out on the first date. And don't fall into that trap of drinking too much and discussing what you did and didn't like about sex with your ex-boyfriend. There won't be much left to the imagination after that conversation. Remember the old saying: Fantasy is often better than reality. Don't give too much away.

So be confident and mysterious. If you feel suddenly insignificant, then cast your mind back to your vast list of achievements and plus points. And remember, the person you're talking to is probably not as confident as they are pretending to be either . . .

Give yourself some inner confidence by wearing fabulous underwear. See IDEA 12, *The power of lovely lingerie.*

Try another idea...

"No one can make you feel inferior without your consent."
ELEANOR ROOSEVELT

Defining idea...

3

How did it go?

Q   What sort of goals are you talking about?

A   *I am talking about small things like doing fifty pelvic floor exercises every day, exfoliating three times a week, or cleaning out your wardrobe. These are not things that one can fail at, since they are not serious, but they keep your mind focused on improving you.*

Q   I can't stop worrying about how I look. Any tips?

A   *Above all, do not fidget. Confident and sexy people do not fidget. They don't need to because they know everything is as it should be. However much you want to whip out that mirror to check your lipstick, hair, false eyelashes—don't. How is anyone going to believe you are the supreme sexual god or goddess of the universe if you don't believe it yourself?*

2

Heaven scent

One of the things that attracts us to each other is smell, or pheromones as we call them in the trade. These are naturally occurring substances that the fertile body secretes externally, sending airborne messages that trigger a response from the opposite sex.

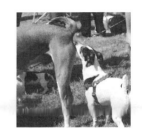

Doubt how important smell is? Think about the person you like the most right now. They walk into a room and come closer. Your heart is beating so hard you can hardly breathe. They bend forward to kiss you and suddenly you're hit with a whiff of body odor. Forget it.

You have to smell good. This is a very basic rule of sex appeal: Clean is a good smell to go for. Too much scent or cologne is off-putting and you don't want to disguise your natural pheromones, those seriously powerful substances men and women emit to attract one another. To make sure you apply your perfume subtly try spraying a little into the air and then walking through the mist rather than spraying the perfume directly onto your body.

Here's an idea for you... **Try putting some scent behind your knees. This is a highly erogenous zone that is often ignored. Don't forget the nape of your neck (a single movement of your head will have him gasping for more) and (women only) between your breasts (the most voluptuous and velvety part of your body—use it).**

In one recent experiment scientists sprayed a chair in a doctor's waiting room with male pheromones (for those of you that are interested, you can buy them on the Internet, some sites even offer a money-back guarantee). A significant proportion of the women who walked into the empty waiting room picked that chair to sit on, despite the fact that it was neither the most comfortable nor the most convenient.

In most animals the relationship between pheromones and mating is pretty basic. Sea urchins, for example, release pheromones into the water surrounding them. Almost immediately other sea urchins eject their sex cells. Ants who meet on a path will pause to rub antennae, thus exchanging pheromones to identify each other. With humans it's usually a little more complicated. But smell is a fundamental factor. If you are looking for the perfect partner, the pheromones in your body scent will play a large part. Dr. Winifred Cutler, a biologist who carried out a lot of work on pheromones in the 1970s, discovered that 74 percent of people who tested a commercially manufactured pheromone experienced an increase in hugging, kissing, and sexual intercourse.

The perception of our body odors is highly subjective; some will find us appealing, others won't. Interestingly, we usually smell best to a person whose genetic immunity to disease differs most from our own. In the long run, this makes for stronger, healthier children.

If you smell something truly disgusting, like rotten eggs, you never forget it. Smells also evoke memories and have been said to do this more vividly than either images or sounds. A friend of mine fell in love with her now husband while in a bath full of expensive bubble bath. "This was fifteen years ago," she tells me, "but we still use the same one if we ever go away for a romantic weekend and the smell takes me back all those years. It reminds me of how crazy we were about each other."

If you smoke, give up—it makes you smell bad. Look at IDEA 13, *Smoke gets in your eyes*, for tips on how to quit.

Try another idea...

Smell is a powerful reminder and an essential ingredient in a relationship. From the first pheromonal attraction to the scent you most associate with your partner, don't underestimate it—when it comes to being incredibly sexy, you need to smell right. Keep clean and select a special scent that for the rest of their life will remind your partner of you. Yes, I told you it was important. Don't just throw on any old scent that Aunt Susan gave you for Christmas. Take an afternoon to explore and experiment in your nearest department store, getting an idea of what fragrances you like and those you don't. It is your signature scent and you want it to reflect your personality.

"You may break, you may shatter the vase, if you will, But the scent of roses will hang round it still."
THOMAS MOORE

Defining idea...

7

How did it go?

Q **I am amazed by the number of scents on the market. How do I choose?**

A *The first thing to do is to ask an expert. Go into a shop and tell them the sort of thing you're after. If it's clean and fresh, then White Linen by Estée Lauder might be the one. If it's mystery you're after, try Sicily by Dolce & Gabbana. There are a few tips when shopping for scent. First, don't wear any. Second, don't try more than three on at any one time. Third, don't buy it the same day; get a tester and try it for several days. And finally, go shopping for scent in the morning, when your senses are heightened.*

Q **I can't tell one aftershave from another. How do I choose one?**

A *Again, you need to decide on the image you want to portray. Classic? Go for Eau Sauvage by Yves Saint Laurent. Something a little less conservative? Try the citrus-based Givenchy Pour Homme. Looking for a masculine image? Polo Sport by Ralph Lauren. As with the scents, you need to go aftershave shopping in the morning and not try too many on at once. But the easiest and most effective thing might just be to let her choose what turns her on.*

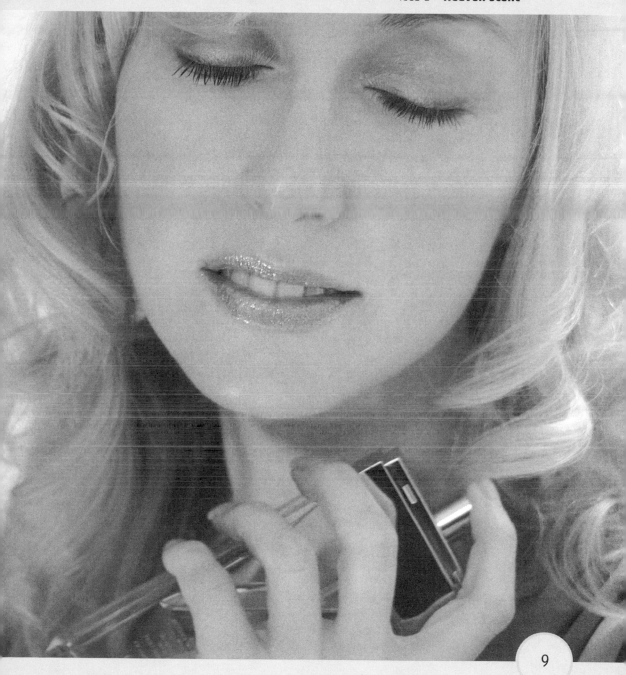

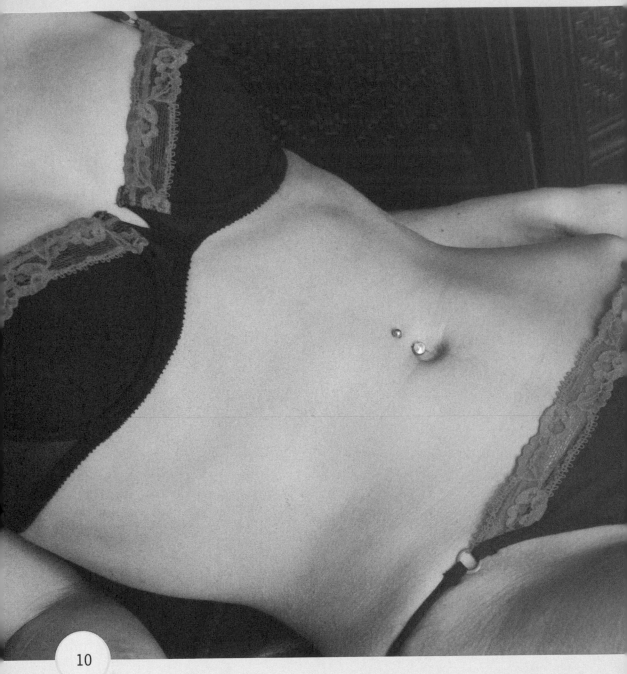

3

A good dressing-down

Less is sometimes more but, conversely, when it comes to looking sexy, flesh is sometimes less. Learn the art of leaving something to the imagination.

There's nothing as off-putting as someone who is trying too hard to look sexy. And the easiest way to do this is to dress "too young" when we've left twenty-five far behind.

Sex appeal has a lot to do with confidence. My aunt, a very chic Italian lady, always told me as a gawky teenager to try to look a bit more frivolous. She would casually throw a shawl over my shoulders and tell me to "carry it." At the time I had no idea what she was talking about. Now I understand that she was trying to get me to wear clothes in a sexy manner, to ooze confidence and frivolity.

So how does one do it? The first thing is not to wear anything uncomfortable. It's very hard to look oh-so-cool if your bra is digging into your ribs. Second, don't wear anything too risky. The skirt riding up to reveal a red thong is not a classy look. I once wore one of those T-shirts with huge holes for the arms that were all the rage

Here's an idea for you... **Go commando. Going out without wearing your underwear makes you feel amazingly sexy. And it's a secret only you know—until you decide to share it with your partner of course . . .**

in the '80s. As I walked down the entire length of a bus, I noticed the whole, totally packed bus staring at me. "I must be looking particularly hot today," I thought to myself. It wasn't until I got off the bus that I noticed the T-shirt was halfway across my chest. And in those days I didn't wear a bra. Another equally devastating incident came when I went on my first date with a demi-god whom I had been lusting after for months. As I put my arms back to let the maître d' take my coat, both my thigh-high stockings fell to my ankles. Great start. So, safety first, wear stuff you know won't embarrass you.

You may be tempted to underdress. And by that I mean wearing something so short it may as well not be there, thinking this looks sexy. Although men like a woman to be in touch with her inner tramp, most don't necessarily want the rest of the world to see their date looking like a lap dancer. The look you need to master is sexy but classy—chic and elegant with a hint of raunchy for the girls, and well turned out at all times for the guys. (Personally, I find pink shirts irresistible, but others may not.)

If your twenties have come and gone it is essential to avoid the mutton-dressed-as-lamb look. If you are over forty, be proud of it. There is no reason why you can't be sexy, but think refined and subtle like Audrey Hepburn.

This idea of having a model in your mind when you shop is a useful one. Before investing in those sequined trousers ask yourself whether your icon would wear them.

Go for that chic French look with **IDEA 43**, *A certain je ne sais quoi.*

Try another idea...

The way clothes feel to the touch is also important, especially if you're aiming for body contact, so think about wearing clothes that follow the contours of your body and that are made of sensual fabrics such as silk, cashmere, velvet, mohair, chiffon, and chenille.

There is such a lot of choice out there and the way you dress will make a huge difference in how you feel, how you sit in a chair, how you walk down the street. Which in turn determines how sexy you'll be.

"Clothes maketh the man."
EARLY 15TH-CENTURY PROVERB

Defining idea...

How did it go?

Q   I don't really know what looks good on me, and I make too many fashion errors. How can I avoid them?

A   *Go to a big department store and hire a professional shopper to advise you. This will cost a bit of money but you only need to do it once and then you can take her advice with you on every shopping trip you ever make. You'll probably find that your shopper chooses things for you that you would never have gone for yourself. This can be very liberating and transform your view about what you can and should wear.*

Q   I am always unsure of the sort of image I will project. I have a hot date coming up and want to make a good first impression—can you help?

A   *There are a couple of basic rules. If you wear light colors you will come across as more innocent and vulnerable. If you wear bold colors you will seem in charge. Think about your date—what would appeal to him? If you want to look sexy but in a completely unobvious way, then wear clothes that if he were to undress you would guide him; for example a shirt with buttons down the front or a dress with a zipper all the way down the back. Men find the thought of what is underneath the zipper or buttons intriguing.*

4

Dance yourself sexy

Dancing is described as the vertical expression of a horizontal desire. And we automatically assume that a good dancer is a good lover.

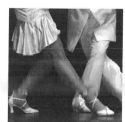

There is nothing quite as sexy as someone who dances well. A body moving gracefully and in time to music is a joy to behold.

Some lunatic flying around a dance floor is not. Think of the film *Dirty Dancing*—would Patrick Swayze have seemed so attractive if he didn't have those dance moves up his sleeve? *Saturday Night Fever* did the same thing for John Travolta—although watching it now he looks slightly ridiculous. So how do you become a sexy dancer? It has a lot to do with rhythm. And relaxing. It's rare to see a man who can dance well. The only one I have ever known was a professional. He was very cute as well, but his dancing put him on another level.

One way to increase your chances on the dance floor is to go back to basics. You may not want to learn ballroom dancing or the foxtrot, but if you have the basic steps you're halfway there. There are lots of Internet sites offering to teach people to dance, so you don't even have to leave your own home as you struggle through

Here's an idea for you...

Become a lap dancer in the privacy of your own home. It's easy to learn how. Search for online tips or rent movies featuring stripping such as *Striptease* **and** *Showgirls*. **It's fairly straightforward though: Just dance seductively wearing very little while your partner/audience stuffs cash into your thong; sexy, fun,** *and* **profitable. Some exercise classes now use pole dancing as a way to get fit. Check out Polestars, which has a great website.**

the first stages. Or you could go straight for a belly dancing course (also available online) and wow your partner with your technique.

Most people would agree that the sexiest dances are those from Latin America. If you have the chance to go to tango or samba classes nearby then go for it. You don't have to live in Rio to samba. It is the most accessible of dances and everyone loves the energetic music. Join up with a local class and get those moves going. If you don't feel like going to a class buy a DVD that teaches you how to samba and rope your partner (roommate, grandma, postman, etc.) in so you can learn together. You'll be amazed at how those hips start to loosen up on the dance floor once you have a few moves under your belt.

Dance classes are a great thing to do together. You'll learn a lot of good moves together that will give your relationship a boost, not to mention making you a total hit on the dance floor. It takes very little to look very good. Even if you're not a natural dancer a few choice moves will make you look truly professional and competent. Find music you really enjoy and this will give you added enjoyment, whether it be salsa or rock 'n' roll.

You need to be fit to dance. Try IDEA 11, *Fitting in fitness*, for tips on how to get in shape.

Try another idea...

If you don't have time to take classes before your next appearance on the dance floor try these tips to make you look cool:

- Relax—let the rhythm flow over you. There is nothing worse than a tense dancer.

- Don't do too much—it's not about how much you move, but how you move.

- Be aware—look around you, not at the floor, be aware of the person you're dancing with, try not to trip over them, stand on their toes, etc.

"Dance is the hidden language of the soul."
MARTHA GRAHAM, modern dancer and choreographer

Defining idea...

How did it go?

Q **I just get so embarrassed dancing with someone. It feels all unnatural and I don't know where to look. What can I do?**

A *Relax—they're probably feeling the same way. Look at them, smile, let the rhythm flow over you, think about the fact that dancing is an advertisement for what might come later—don't waste it.*

Q **I feel so silly asking a girl to dance these days. Is it even politically correct to ask?**

A *Political correctness, how tedious, eh? Since when did a girl not want to be treated like a princess? We all grow up listening to the same fairy tales and we all want the happy ending. If you ask a girl nicely (think Mr. Darcy not Eminem) and she says no, she is either having a bad day or you're not her type. But she will still be grateful that you asked. I defy any girl to tell me she no longer wants to be wooed.*

5

And what do you do?

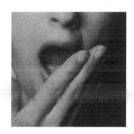

Small talk. Hideous. My idea of hell is standing around a cocktail party while people ask me what I do. I know that it's a useful question for generating fifteen further minutes of conversation. But it's right up there with, "Do you come here often?" in the tedium stakes as a first line.

Being sexy is not just about the way you look, smell, and dress. It's about your character. One word that people associate with sexy is "enigmatic" so try to make your first line something a bit more unusual.

In the film *White Mischief*, Charles Dance checks out Greta Scacchi as they walk down the stairs. There is an obvious magnetism between them. At the bottom of the stairs he turns to her and says, "Are you going to tell your husband, or shall I?"

OK, that's fantasy, not reality. But it certainly beats, "What do you do?" in the first line stakes. I remember my father telling me off when I was about twelve for saying I was hungry. "Don't be so banal," he said. "Use your imagination. Instead of saying

Here's an idea for you...

Jerry Hall once suggested wives should read something interesting every day so that when their husbands returned from work they had something interesting to talk about. Old-fashioned but we can all learn from the principle. If you don't do, read, see, or experience anything new, you're not going to have much to talk about. So try to stay well-informed and alert; it's much sexier than ignorant.

you're hungry say: 'The people in the street seem to me transformed into plates of pasta coming toward me.' " OK, so he is Italian—and crazy—but get the idea? Think slightly eccentric, quirky, and charming. Instead of coming out with a line people expect you to say, dare to be different. Try starting with something that happened to you recently, or something interesting you've read or seen in the news. The conversation will flow from whatever starting point you give it, but the person's impression of you will be different.

I can't remember the number of times I have been stuck next to people at dinner parties and they have started talking about commuting or childcare. Deadly. At first I wondered whether it was me. Was I really so dull that all people could find to talk to me about was that? But when I compared notes with friends they said they'd experienced the same thing. I resolved to counterattack. Every time someone started to talk about either topic I would say, "Isn't it extraordinary how as soon as we get to a dinner party we start to talk about nannies or commuting? I'd much rather talk about sex, wouldn't you?" Either they start to bore the person on their other side or you can get into a gritty sexy conversation. Marvelous! Changing the tack of the conversation is good practice and just as valuable as avoiding being a dull conversationalist yourself.

Most people like to talk about themselves and have something interesting to say, even if it's not immediately apparent. In other words, you need to bring this something interesting out of them. Remember that you can learn something from everyone. Even if they initially come across as the dullest person you've ever met, try to use the time with them to bring out their best side.

Check out IDEA 45, *Be a culture vulture*, on how to be interestingly intellectual.

Try another idea...

A good answer to the question, "How old are you?" is, "About your age." This totally floors people and also means you can avoid telling them. Adopt this attitude when people try to make dull conversation. Conversation is a little bit like a sport: You will play to the level you find yourself. If someone is deadly dull, you're more likely to be so yourself and dull is NOT sexy. Either walk away from them or try to change the subject matter. Most people are just as interested as you are to enjoy life. They will also want to sparkle and a good conversation will help them do that. There is nothing more infuriating than watching someone else have a great conversation while you're stuck next to great bores of today talking about trains. Now that you've read this, you need never go there again.

Someone totally intent on talking about trains will not be interested in spending time with the new super-sexy conversationalist you're going to become. You need never be on the periphery of the party again.

"Talking and eloquence are not the same: to speak, and to speak well, are two things."
BEN JOHNSON, 17th-century dramatist and wit

Defining idea...

How did it go?

Q   I just can't talk about sex at a dinner party.

A   *Take it slowly, don't try anything too radical. You don't have to talk about sex, but you don't have to be boring either. Drop in interesting snippets you've picked up from TV, or from reading magazines, as and when you feel comfortable. A good tip for men is to bone up on pop psychology magazines such as Psychology Today as they are chock-full of the sort of interesting psychological insights into how women tick that we enjoy. Above all, relax. What's the worst thing that can happen? The person you're making small talk with will think you're slightly different? Good!*

Q   I wonder if it's possible that some days one just feels boring and others one doesn't?

A   *Of course, some days the original one-liners will just flow. On others you'll feel totally stuck and unable even to tell someone what time it is. If you happen to be out on such a day, don't despair. You will just have to concentrate a bit harder to come across as sexy and amusing. Make an effort. Once you start entertaining yourself, your mood will change.*

6

Sexy mama

Some women see being pregnant as an excuse not to have sex. Madness. Sex when you're pregnant is fantastic. And you can look eye-poppingly sexy, too.

I once went to a party where I saw a heavily pregnant woman who was wearing a very simple black dress. She looked amazing—better than all the other women there. She was elegant, glowing, and beautiful.

Pregnant women have been taught to hide their bump and stay at the back of the crowd until the baby has come out. Things are rapidly changing; there are whole shops dedicated to pregnant women, devoted to making you look good. I loved being pregnant. I was careful not to put on excess weight, but I think there's nothing quite as lovely as a beautiful bump dressed well. And staying sexy while pregnant will make your whole pregnancy experience more enjoyable.

Here's an idea for you...

Rather than hiding your bump, accentuate it. A very chic way to do this is to wrap a brightly colored scarf around it and tie it in a knot to one side. Or wear a short T-shirt and low-cut maternity jeans or a sarong (obviously only when it's warm outside!). Try a lovely slinky (stretchy) dress that hugs the contours of your bump, but make sure it's comfortable—it's very hard to feel sexy when you're focusing on trying to breathe.

The first thing you should remember is that there will come a stage when your normal clothes will not look good anymore. You just have to accept maternity clothes as a fact of life. The specialized maternity shops can be expensive, so try the big department stores, many of which have maternity sections; or buy oversized clothes from thrift stores (my favorite hunting ground). You could also try the Internet, where there are lots of websites vying for your business. Some have really glamorous lines that can be purchased online. You should look upon your pregnancy as an opportunity to dress up and show off that bump, not hide it. I promise, lots of men find it really sexy, and your partner certainly will.

So, sex and the pregnant woman. The first thing to say is that it is perfectly safe for you and your baby. I don't advise swinging from chandeliers as you go into the third trimester, but most things are admissible. It is also a good excuse to experiment with some new positions.

There are several positions for pregnant women that are both comfortable and safe. So if you haven't already tried them, go for it.

Dancing is great exercise for pregnant women—check out IDEA 4, *Dance yourself sexy.*

Try another idea...

- Position one: Woman on top. Lower yourself onto your partner, either facing him or facing his feet. Many women find their nipples are incredibly sensitive when they're pregnant, so if you're facing him, make sure he kisses them

- Position two: The classic missionary position obviously doesn't work with a bump, but this one does. You lie on your back, knees drawn back with your feet resting on your partner's chest, or with your legs straight up and resting against your partner (a good hamstring stretch this one). Your partner kneels between your legs to enter you, so there is no weight on your stomach. You might find it more comfortable with a pillow under your bottom.

- Position three: Side by side. You and your partner lie side by side, facing each other. You can drape your leg over your partner's body. This is not really very practical in the third trimester as the bump gets in the way.

- Position four: Spooning, on the other hand, works throughout. You lie on your side, in a curled position. Your partner lies behind you and enters you from behind. Penetration is shallow, so this can be a comfortable position during late pregnancy.

"Everything you see I owe to spaghetti."
SOPHIA LOREN

■ Position five: From behind. You are on all fours on the bed (or wherever), leaning down onto pillows with your partner kneeling and entering you from behind. Or, try bending over the bed (supported by pillows) with your partner standing and entering from behind. This is what is medically termed a maximum penetration position, so do tell your partner if it gets painful.

■ Position six: Sitting. In this position, you straddle your partner while he is sitting on a sturdy, comfortable chair or on the edge of the bed. You can also sit in an armchair, upright or leaning back slightly, with your legs around your partner, who is kneeling in front of you.

And you thought being pregnant signaled the end of your sex life? There will be no closing up shop early now. Remember, good sex will make you feel and look sexier.

Q **I thought sex when you're pregnant was bad for you. Isn't it a bit disrespectful toward the baby?**

How did it go?

A *Get a grip. I remember when I had orgasms during pregnancy, the baby would do a little somersault and my whole tummy would tighten into a mini-contraction. It was a wonderful feeling. Remember that if you're happy then so is your baby. The chemicals released during orgasm relax you and make you happy. That inner peace is transmitted to your baby. Don't forget that you have a relationship to maintain, as well as a baby to carry. The little newborn wants to come into a good relationship that is alive in every sense.*

Q **I am now about to pop—the thought of intercourse is just too much. What other options are there?**

A *Don't forget, sex is not just about intercourse. Try oral sex, mutual masturbation, massaging, and so on.*

7

Literal appeal

Use books to boost your own sex appeal. Model yourself on your sexiest literary hero or heroine—figure out what makes him or her so attractive and emulate it.

Heathcliff was the first love of my life. I read Wuthering Heights at about age fifteen and fell in love with the swarthy, brooding hero.

When I was at college I read *Riders, Rivals,* and *Polo* and fell deeply in love with Rupert Campbell-Black, Jilly Cooper's most successful and irresistible creation. These men, much more than old boyfriends, have stayed with me forever. I'm sure I was attracted to my husband in part because he's named Rupert. In college I had a series of totally doomed relationships with Byronic (and some might add moronic) characters.

So why is it that we love a literary hero? It has to be said I am not the only adolescent to fall in love with Heathcliff. It is easy to fall in love with a character in a book. You can attribute any qualities you like to them. You have a lot to do with the way they look as well. So what makes a sexy hero or heroine? A lot of the same things that apply to real people. Intelligence, charm, mystery, and charisma. But there is often an element of cruelty, too: The cad seems to do well in literature.

Here's an idea for you...

Have a themed dinner party and allocate a romantic literary hero or heroine to all your guests. By playing a role rather than having to be yourself you'll be able to lose some of your inhibitions and let your sexy side shine through. And who knows, you might find your roommate's brother or the guy from number 42 a lot more interesting when he's dressed up as Rhett Butler!

Take Rochester, the hero of *Jane Eyre*. Although he comes off as good in the end, the facts are he has a wife hidden in the attic and is incredibly bad-tempered. Rupert Campbell-Black is a cad personified; he lies and cheats his way into every bed in the county. Eugene Onegin, the hero in Pushkin's poem of the same name, throws Tatiana's innocent love back in her face. These are men most of us would run a mile from in real life, but from the safety of the living room chair we can fantasize about these passionate types.

So in literature the brooding, Byronic, sometimes Gothic hero rules. In terms of heroines, the sexy ones are harder to define. Ellen Olenska, for example, in Edith Wharton's *The Age of Innocence*, is vulnerable, incredibly beautiful, and on the road to perdition. This seems to be a pattern heroines follow; just consider Anna Karenina, Emma Bovary, Lara Antipova in *Dr. Zhivago*, Tess in *Tess of the D'Urbervilles*, and you'll see what I mean. So in summary, the men are strong (with a hint of evil) and brooding, the women doomed and beautiful. Too clichéd for words but in order to attract a lover, projecting a hint of these qualities wouldn't go amiss.

However, once a relationship is established, you'll be on safer ground using great literary scenarios to create your own passionate moments. Emma Bovary is seduced in the back of a carriage. A carriage might be hard to find, but you shouldn't experience too much difficulty in finding an enclosed space that feels dangerous and risqué. Just make sure you aren't anywhere you're likely to get into trouble—the supermarket parking lot on a Saturday afternoon is probably not a good idca!

Check out IDEA 37, *Absence makes the heart grow fonder*, for tips on how you can woo someone with words.

Try another idea...

The secret is to search out the essence of the sexiness in your chosen book and then apply it to your life. If you feel like a bit of roughness, then read *Lady Chatterley's Lover* by D. H. Lawrence. The aristocratic madamc cnds up having wild sex with a servant—using that as your blueprint could lead to all manner of sexy scenarios.

In *A Room with a View* by E. M. Forster, the hero takes the heroine in his arms and surprises her with a passionate kiss in a field outside Florence. One of the first kisses in modern literature, it is passionate and unexpected. Try to re-create your own impulsive moments, whether you've been married for twenty years or have just met. And don't underestimate the importance of fooling around. Married couples scem to forget all about necking; it's a crucial part of a relationship and should be practiced as often as possible.

"Sex is more exciting on the screen and between the pages than between the sheets."
ANDY WARHOL

Defining idea...

How did it go?

Q **The problem I find is that men in books are much more interesting than men in real life. What can I do?**

A *Not much, I'm afraid. Mr. Darcy is unlikely to come stomping around the corner in his frilly shirt. That's the difference between reality and fantasy. When you finally come across one that is better than the fantasy, you've found your Mr. Right. Until then, keep reading and dreaming.*

Q **All this literature is great, but I don't really get a charge out of reading. How can I develop an interest?**

A *Maybe you're going for the wrong kind of books? You could try audio books until you get the flavor of them. You can rent them from your local library and they're great company when you're out jogging or walking the dog. If all this fails and it's erotic literature you really want, then read the French porn classic Emmanuelle. My husband never travels without his copy and as soon as he hears someone is named Emmanuelle, he gets terribly excited. Sad, really.*

8

White hot wedding

It's the most important day of your life. You want to look totally incredible, better than you've ever looked before and sexier as well.

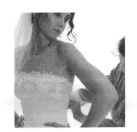

Everything has to work: the makeup, the hair, the shoes, the underwear, and most importantly, for the bride, the dress.

But first you need to decide what sort of bride you want to be. If you're over thirty-five and getting married for the second time the pure white virgin look is just plain silly. When I got married I went for the movie star look. The dress looked like something worn by Kim Basinger in *L.A. Confidential* and made me feel as sexy as she was in that film. When I got to the altar my husband-to-be told me I looked like a movie star. This was a good start to married life and exactly the reaction you want.

You need to look wonderful. You don't want to look like you look every other day but you also need to be careful about not veering too far away from your true character. You don't want to be totally unrecognizable. The dress is really the single most important thing in the whole wedding preparation. More than anything on the day, the dress is going to define you, set up your image, and give off the vibes you want to project.

Here's an idea for you...

Pay huge attention to the detail in your wedding outfit, especially the shoes. Nothing lets an image down quite as much as cheap finishing touches. Make sure the flowers in your hair and your bouquet are the best. This is not a time to be saving $10 here and there.

So where to start looking? Leafing through magazines will save a lot of traipsing around, and check out the Internet as well. If you see an amazing dress in a magazine that is way above your budget, why not see if you can get someone to make a copy of it for you?

So, you have a dress that is sexy and suitable but what about the rest? First of all, there's your hair, which above all needs to be comfortable. You'll find it incredibly irritating and distracting if you constantly need to fiddle with the do. If it is long, put it up and leave it alone. Wearing a veil is a strange sensation and one you're unlikely to repeat unless you take holy orders, so you need to get used to it beforehand. Wander around the yard for a few hours wearing it; that'll get the neighbors talking. Your makeup needs to be flawless all day, because you'll be on show, so get one of your bridesmaids to regularly monitor how you're looking. Needless to say, on an emotional day like this you'll need waterproof eye makeup. And finally, your underwear—you'll probably want this to be the sexiest underwear you've ever had but just remember that you'll be wearing it for a long time, so it needs to be comfortable, too.

Obviously being a sexy bride is also about how you feel and not just how you look. However, your look will, of course, boost your confidence and therefore sexiness. But your attitude and mood are also hugely important. Try to delegate as much of the running of the day as possible so you can focus on being yourself and enjoying what is *your* day. And of course, night. The wedding night is not as big a deal as it was 100 years ago, when it was the first time you saw a naked man, but still, it is an important milestone. It is the first time you are sleeping together as man and wife, which in itself will make the whole event sexier. Try to stay relatively sober (I wish I had) so you can at least remember it in the morning. Making love to your new husband wearing nothing but a wedding ring and a garter belt will be the perfect end to a perfect day.

If you're stuck for ideas on where to go for your honeymoon take a look at IDEA 34, *Wow, voyager!*

Try another idea…

"I chose my wife, as she did her wedding gown, not for a fine glossy surface, but such qualities as would wear well."
OLIVER GOLDSMITH

Defining idea…

Q   I want to look like a natural beauty on my wedding day. How do I get the non-made-up look but still make the best of my face?

A   *One option is to employ a makeup artist. It costs a bit but it is only for one day. Or do what I did and go to the makeup counter in your local department store, tell them you're getting married, and get them to do a mini makeover on the spot. Most places won't charge you for the makeover providing you then buy the products. If you take a piece of material from your wedding dress with you, they can match the nails and lipstick to it.*

Q   If I don't go for white, what are the other options?

A   *Cream is an obvious choice, or go for gold as I did (sounds terrible but it was great). For something different why not go for the ethnic boho chic look, although something slightly more classic might be less of an embarrassment in forty years' time. If you're getting married at the courthouse then you could go for a classic suit in a pale color. The only thing to avoid is black.*

9

The art of the sexy surprise

Everyday married or cohabiting life can get dull. Sex just isn't what it used to be. The spice has gone out of the relationship. It comes back now and again, but is more evident by its absence.

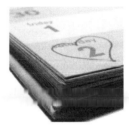

We all remember the initial excitement of the first hot date, the first kiss, and the first time you ever woke up together. The tragedy is that the ecstasy doesn't last forever.

We soon fall into familiar patterns of life that don't necessarily include mind-blowing passion and wild sex. This is where surprises are so important. I'm not talking about presents, but about things that ignite your sexual relationship or, if you're about to start a relationship, things that will bring results.

Here then is a top-ten list of sexy actions. Don't try them all at once!

1. After a sedate dinner (once the kids have gone to bed) tell your partner that dessert is on you. Literally. Get the ice cream and spread it all over.

Here's an idea for you...

Why not treat your loved one to a day at a spa? Enjoy all the facilities offered: sauna, Jacuzzi, and pool. Just focus on yourselves and your bodies for twenty-four hours. What could be better than that? Once back in your room, try out some of the massage techniques you've experienced on each other.

2. Go to dinner at your in-laws' wearing no underwear. But be sure to let him know you're not wearing any just as you get out of the car. He can mull over the fact all through dinner and ravish you on your way home.

3. Rent a porn movie. Nothing too drastic. Watch it together with a bottle of champagne.

4. Go to bed in garters and stockings on what is otherwise a normal weekday. Obviously you need to make sure he sees them! So saunter oh-so-casually past him to get a glass of water or turn on the alarm clock.

5. Go to a sex shop together. You don't need to buy the double-headed black mamba, for heaven's sake. In fact, some sex shops now are perfectly respectable places to be seen in. And you never know what you might find.

6. Fantasize—you can do this together and it works well. Imagine you're somewhere or someone else.

7. Pounce—this will obviously only work if you're alone in the house. Pick your moment and pounce on him or her. The unexpected approach will be a huge turn-on. Just make sure it's somewhere less obvious than the bedroom. Go for the bathroom or the kitchen table. Remember that scene in *The Postman Always Rings Twice?* Jack Nicholson and Jessica Lange covered in flour and consumed with passion.

   Surprise your lover with a sexy fantasy—see IDEA 30, *Sex on the brain*.

   Try another idea...

8. Sex slaves—promise to be his or her sex slave for the next two hours.

9. Promise him oral sex whenever he wants it. The generosity of this gift will touch any man. And amaze most of them. The most common complaint about their sex life I hear from my male friends is that they never get oral sex from their partners.

10. Check out a new position on the Internet or in a book and try it out on him or her. But be careful about looking at porn on the web and never leave your name and email address.

"Life is a great surprise."
VLADIMIR NABOKOV

Defining idea...

How did it go?

Q **What if my advances are rejected? What if he calls me a slut for going to his parents' house with no underwear on?**

A *If he does that you should put your underwear firmly over his head and leave. But you do need to gauge what your partner will like or how far he or she will comfortably want to go. It is unlikely if you've picked up this book that you're a complete prude and therefore I assume that your partner won't be either. But be aware that he or she may have limits that you may have to wear down slowly.*

Q **I'm too tired for all of this. How can I muster up some energy?**

A *I know that feeling. All you want to do is collapse into bed and you'd be asleep before he's gotten your garters off. Try to pick a time when you're not exhausted. And if you simply don't have any time then you will just have to sacrifice something else. What could be more important than keeping your relationship alive and spicy?*

10

Work it!

This is the idea you need when you have to be smart and sassy at 8 a.m. and gorgeous and sexy at 8 p.m. and there is no time to go home in between.

You can't quite believe it's happened. The man of your dreams (and we're talking fairly graphic dreams) has finally asked you out on a date.

Great news. The bad news is that you have a hugely important presentation that day, followed by a client lunch, and then a data training session all afternoon. There is no time to go home and freshen up between work and play.

Don't panic. The first thing to do is to start your preparation early. The night before go to bed early, having had a long bath, done your nails, waxed your legs, plucked your eyebrows, and so forth. Get into bed wearing a moisturizing mask (my favorites are the really thick and creamy ones). Don't take it off but leave it on all night—believe me, it's worth the messy pillowcase in the morning.

The next morning take a shower, wash your hair, and prepare yourself as you normally would for a day at work. The key is in what you take with you to work.

Here's an idea for you...

Take another pair of shoes to the office to change into for the evening. There's nothing quite as refreshing as taking off shoes you have been running around in all day.

I am guessing you will have at least an hour between leaving work and the date. This time needs to be used to give you that "just left the bathroom" look and feel. To achieve this you will have to bring to the office makeup remover, face moisturizer, toothbrush, hairbrush, scent, deodorant, new underwear, tights/stockings, and a change of clothes. Some little extras could include a product that promises to brighten up your face like a beauty flash balm—most makeup companies do one (but be sure to apply makeup right away afterward or it flakes).

Once you have finished your high-powered day, lock yourself in the ladies' bathroom. If the one at the office isn't very nice then be bold: Walk to the nearest luxury hotel and march into theirs. If you walk in looking confident, people rarely question you. The downside to changing outside the office is that you will have to carry your old work clothes with you all night.

Once in a bathroom, remove day makeup and immediately apply your moisturizer. Then wash under your arms (amazing how much fresher you will feel if you do this); if you can, also wash your feet. People may come in wondering what on earth you're on, but if you want to smell and look good for the man of your dreams do you really care if you end up with a reputation for being a bit quirky?

Once you're washed, brush your teeth, apply your makeup, then change your clothes, brush your hair, spray on some scent, and you're ready. If you have about half an hour and your date is in a town or city, you might want to pop into a hairdresser's for a quick wash and blow-dry. Then you can do your makeup there. But you should probably get the underarm and feet washing out of the way beforehand!

If you have more time on your hands, go for a full preparation technique. See IDEA 48, *Preparation, preparation, preparation*.

Try another idea...

So that's the way you look dealt with. Now for your psyche: You need to shake away the office from your brain as well as your body. If you can find somewhere you're unlikely to be disturbed, a good way to do this is to do some gentle stretching exercises. Stand up straight, reach your arms above your head, and then breathe out as you reach for your toes. Breathe in once you're down there and clasp your ankles. Slowly breathe in as you bend you knees and breathe out as you straighten them, edging closer to the floor with each breath. Repeat this ten times and ignore any stressful thoughts that try to crowd your brain. Next, raise your arms above your head, breathing out as you go up. Breathe in as you slowly lower your arms to your side. Repeat five times. Remember to focus on where you're going, who you're meeting, and what you want out of the date . . . the office can wait until tomorrow.

"Be prepared."
MOTTO OF THE BOY SCOUTS OF AMERICA

Defining idea...

How did it go?

Q **How will I stay perky after a really busy day?**

A *You'd be amazed what adrenaline does for you. A friend of mine recently had a hugely important date after a horrendous day that started with an overnight flight from New York, meetings all day, and lunch with her boss. But the excitement of the date kept her going and by midnight she had so much adrenaline rushing around her system (along with some alcohol) that she was positively radiant. If you can't rely on natural adrenaline give your system a helping hand by downing some effervescent vitamin C tablets.*

Q **Anything else I can do to freshen up?**

A *You could take some breath fresheners with you and pop one in just a few minutes before you're due to meet. You can cut out the full change of clothes and just take another shirt or top with you. If you're a man you might want to think about at least bringing another pair of socks. Don't forget to dispose of the others somewhere though; you don't want her to come across them while seductively caressing you.*

11

Fitting in fitness

No one wants to go to bed with a slob. The biological basis of sex appeal dictates that we find fit-looking people more attractive.

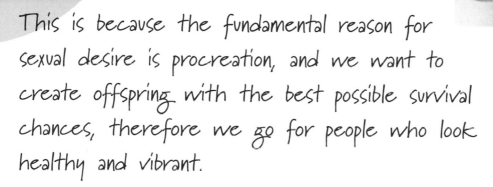

This is because the fundamental reason for sexual desire is procreation, and we want to create offspring with the best possible survival chances, therefore we go for people who look healthy and vibrant.

So it's time to dust off the Stairmaster and get those buttocks working—here's how to boost your sex appeal and self-image by thinking about your body all day long.

Get into the habit of doing a ten-minute exercise routine as soon as you get up. This involves 100 sit-ups, 50 lunges (stand up with legs together, stride one foot forward and bend the knee, then come back up to the starting position and do the same with the other leg) on each leg, 25 push-ups (on your knees or against a wall if you can't do full ones), and some stretching. The sit-ups should be a mixture of two very different techniques. First, 25 of your normal crunches. Then rest on your arms while you raise both legs together, slowly, until they are about a foot and a half from the

Here's an idea for you...

Try these easy push-ups. Stand facing a wall with your arms shoulder-width apart. With hands on the wall, slowly fall toward it and then push yourself back with your arms. Repeat this 35 times. It's a great way to keep the upper body in shape without falling flat on your face while trying to do a push-up.

floor. Then lower them, even more slowly. Repeat this 25 times. If you can't feel it, you're either blessed with a washboard stomach or not doing it right. Try lying flat on your back and doing the same thing—it's a killer. Now do 25 crunches where you bring your legs and top half of the body together, thus working the lower abdominals, and finally another 25 leg raises (try one leg at a time if you can't face both together). The lunges can be varied with alternative buttock clenches. Lie on your back with your legs bent and hip-width apart. Raise your buttocks, squeezing them as you go up, and simultaneously bring your knees together.

After you've completed the routine, brush your body all over before taking a shower—once you're clean, turn the water to cold and stay put for ten seconds. Sounds terrifying, but you'll get used to it. I was brought up in Scandinavia and there we thought nothing of running from a steaming hot sauna to throw ourselves headfirst into the snow.

So now you're set up for the day. Walk to the subway/bus/car clenching your butt as you go. At first this will make you walk strangely, but keep it up. At the office, shun the elevator (unless the man of your dreams is in there) and run up the stairs (two at a time if you're feeling really fit). You'll arrive breathless but with better buttocks. Throughout the day, hold in your stomach. You'll look instantly better and it's great for stomach tone. Keep clenching your butt whenever you can. In other words, just squeeze everything at all times.

Stuck in a line? Don't get irritated while you're waiting; use the time to clench and squeeze. If you're on the subway or the train and it grinds to a standstill think "yippee, some time to do some subtle butt exercises" and start squeezing for all you're worth. Hold for thirty seconds, relax, and start again.

Now that you're fit, check out IDEA 52, *Anyone for tennis?*, for sexy hobbies to try.

Try another idea...

Never waste a minute in your quest for a sexy body—and you can work the inside as well as the outside. When I became pregnant for the first time I asked my yoga teacher about pelvic floor exercises. This is the little muscle you squeeze if you want to stop your pee from coming out. When you have babies it gets stretched and you need to be very careful not to let it get out of shape. You could find yourself incontinent, or even worse, unable to enjoy sex. I was expecting her to tell me to do around 100 a day. "Do one big one," she said. "Start it when you wake up in the morning and stop when you go to sleep at night!" So, if you're ever bored with someone's conversation, use the time to *squeeze* that pelvic floor—pretend you're trying to stop peeing mid-flow. Hold it. Let go. Repeat (as often as you possibly can). As you get better at it, try to increase the pressure of the squeezes, but if you are in mid-conversation make sure you don't scrunch up your face at the same time.

"It is better to be looked over than overlooked."
MAE WEST

Defining idea...

Q   **I feel so fat and unhealthy; just the thought of exercising fills me with dread. How can I get going?**

A   *You'd be amazed how quickly things improve. The first few times will feel tough but then you'll start to get addicted to the feeling you get from the exercise and the results. It's all a question of attitude. Like one of those awful spring cleaning jobs you just can't face starting, it's a lot easier than you imagined it would be, and actually quite good fun.*

Q   **Is there anything simple that I can ease into exercise with?**

A   *You could start power walking. Get decked out so you really feel the part—sexy shorts, T-shirt, and MP3 player full of inspiring music. Or go with a friend and gossip your way around the park. Walk fast, but don't overstride—it's bad for your ligaments. Pump your arms while you're doing it to increase heart rate. Walking briskly uses up as many calories as jogging slowly and it's gentler on your joints. Remember to clench those buttocks as you go. This is great for people who hate the gym. Being outside is a wonderful way of slowing life down—you observe the seasons passing firsthand rather than via a car window. Also, breathing in all that fresh air is great for your skin—just remember to wear sunscreen.*

12

The power of lovely lingerie

Underwear. It's crucial. Get it right and you feel great. It's an essential part of being incredibly sexy.

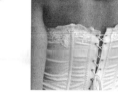

It boosts your confidence and helps you look marvelous in and out of your clothes. What's not to love?

When I first traveled to Europe I was amazed at all the little underwear shops selling lingerie at what I thought were extortionate prices. I reasoned that there was nothing wrong with a pack of five panties for the price of one bra-strap in some fancy store. Up to a point I was right. There are days when those cotton no-frills panties work well. But what is truly different about your average French woman is that she will wear sexy matching bra and panties every day. And she is prepared to spend around $60 on each ensemble.

Now that I live in France I have gone very French in my attitude toward underwear. My bra and underwear drawers are stuffed full of matching ensembles. And oddly enough, once I started doing this, I found it hard to go back to the five-packs. There's something empowering about matching top to bottom and for this reason you should seriously consider buying at least two pairs of underwear with each bra. To

Here's an idea for you...

This expensive underwear is all very well, but a pain to hand wash. I take mine into the shower with me and wash it there, which is much easier. It also means you don't end up with that awful grey shade of white as your delicates get washed on a sixty-degree cycle with all the wrong colors. Treat it well and it will last much longer.

make sure you don't suffer from the dreaded VPL (visible panty line) under trousers always make at least one of these pairs a thong, or try out French panties or boxer shorts for girls—no VPL and damn sexy!

Sex appeal has a lot to do with confidence and there is nothing like good underwear to enhance your body shape and make you feel more attractive. For the flatter-chested among us, there is no more comforting moment than pulling a T-shirt over a new Wonderbra and seeing our body shapes totally transformed. For larger ladies, a good well-fitting bra is even more essential. If you want to minimize your bust under business suits, get measured by an expert to find out your correct cup size—I swear you will lose ten pounds immediately when you put on the right fitting bra. And if you want to emphasize your cleavage, a correctly fitting bra does this stupendously well, besides being much more comfortable.

A sexy thong can work wonders for your butt. Some people find them incredibly uncomfortable—I did to begin with—but once you get used to them you will hardly ever wear ordinary underwear again.

If you're wearing the right underwear, you feel like you can take on the world. It makes you feel so much more confident. You walk into a business meeting and although the others can't see what you've got on underneath your suit, you know, and it gives you a sense of superiority. I spoke to Chantal Thomass, France's leading underwear designer, on this subject. "Lingerie is fundamental to the way a woman feels," she says. "If your underwear isn't right, nothing else works." A friend of mine says it determines her whole mood for the day: "It's the first thing I put on and it puts me in a good or bad mood," she says. "I have a very intimate relationship with my lingerie; after all it is the thing I put on next to my skin."

As we all know, for whatever reason, men *adore* stockings and garters. Just about every man I know is totally crazy for them. "I don't know what it is about them," says one. "They just drive me wild. Maybe it's because all the Playboy models I lusted over in my youth wore them." Our job here is not to analyze; just wear them. Classic black garter belts are the best, but red can be good for a special occasion, adding an extra sex-vixen allure. The great thing about kinky or sexy underwear is that it enhances your sex drive as well as your partner's. You're hardly going to sit around feeling like a slob in a pair of red crotchless panties!

You need to have good skin to best show off your new underwear. Go to IDEA 24, *The art of the sexy bath*, for tips.

Try another idea...

"A lady is one who never shows her underwear unintentionally."
LILLIAN DAY, author

Defining idea...

How did it go?

Q **I don't really have the confidence to go dressing up in strange underwear. What do you suggest?**

A *Who said anything about it having to be strange? You could start with a very classic matching bra and panties. Even if you can't afford La Perla, you should check it out and see if you can find a cheaper version somewhere. It is the most stunning underwear ever and will give you an idea of how crucial underwear can be. If you're wearing a La Perla all-in-one, the sky's the limit. Wolford isn't bad either, and is much cheaper, although still not a steal. Check out the sales—most large department stores stock Wolford. They do great tights and stockings as well, so are well worth looking at. If you look after them (i.e., don't put them in the washing machine) they can last for several years. Check them out at www.wolford.com.*

Q **How about sexy underwear for us guys?**

A *Now you're talking. Amazingly, men are catching up. There are some great websites now offering all sorts of goodies, including the very slinky l'homme invisible. Totally irresistible. There's also a solution for men who feel nature has been a little stingy in the lunch-box department. A website (go find it if you're really interested) is offering two models of padded pants: colt or stallion (oh, please). The blurb promises the padding is discreetly tucked away in hidden pockets and will change your life. Until you take your pants off, that is.*

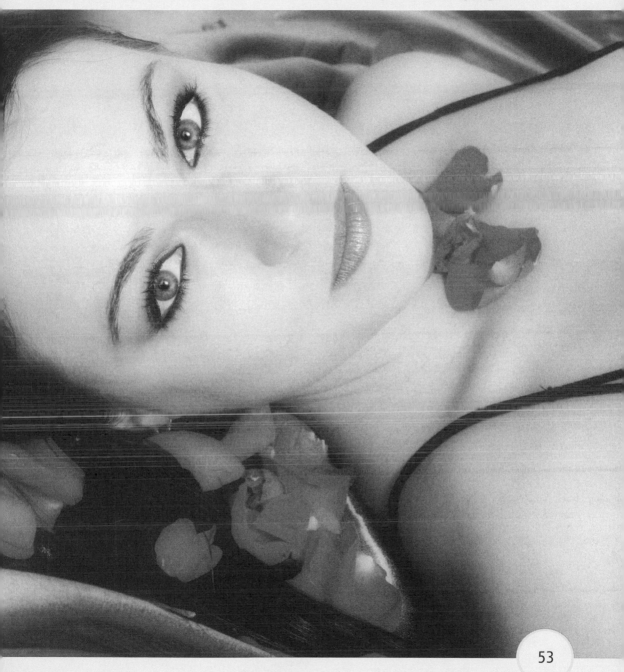

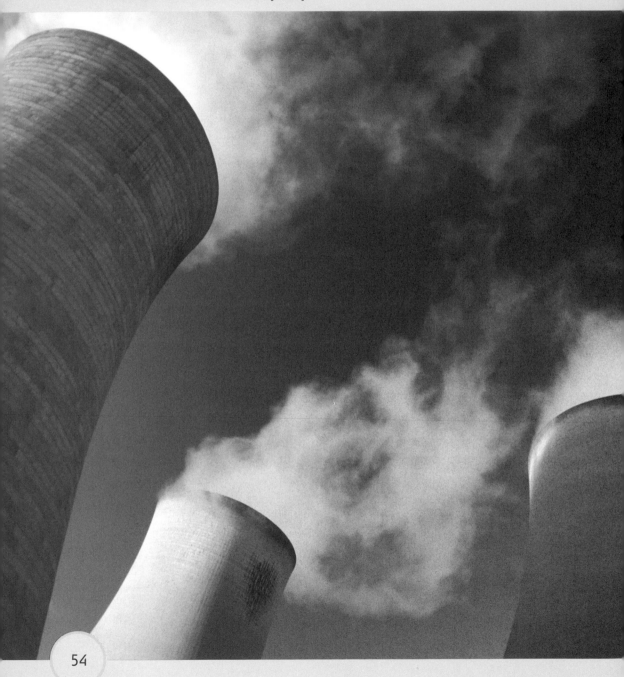

13

Smoke gets in your eyes

It's one of the defining moments of film: Lauren Bacall and Humphrey Bogart. "You know how to whistle, don't you?" she smolders. "You just put your lips together and . . . blow." As she speaks, she exhales a cloud of smoke.

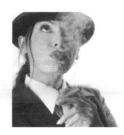

The effect of the smoke is to make her even more mysterious, more seductive. I admit it, Lauren Bacall looked cool and sexy smoking. But you won't.

Sorry to be so blunt about it but there is nothing sexy about smoking nowadays. The underlying reason is very simple. Sex has everything to do with life. Smoking is now associated with death and disease. The two are incompatible. So how to stop? There are countless books about this, which just shows you that most smokers want to quit the habit. First of all, don't underestimate the task. Smoking is harder to quit than heroin. I can't do a compare and contrast but I have given up smoking and it was terribly difficult.

I didn't do it all at once. Instead of smoking all day, I told myself I could only smoke when I went out. The problem with this was that smoking is such a powerful drug that I found myself going out just so I could have a cigarette. Still, it was a start. I

Here's an idea for you...

Every time you want a cigarette, do something else. For example, have a glass of water. It will make you feel fresh, saintly, and won't make your breath smell bad. Prepare a jug first thing in the morning with some slices of lemon and lime, maybe some ice cubes. This is also a good way to stop putting on weight, one of the major downsides of giving up smoking. Hunger pangs are often thirst pangs in disguise.

also allowed myself to smoke in a crisis. Strangely enough, I still have anxiety dreams that I pick up a cigarette in a panic situation and am then back to square one, a miserable addict yet again. And this is fifteen years after I quit.

The most sensible thing to do is to stop altogether, but if you can't, then take it step by step. If you really want to stop you will get there eventually. There are lots of crutches you can use, such as nicotine patches and chewing gum. Speak to your doctor for advice on what might work best for you.

If you feel it's all too much at once then cut down. Go from twenty one day to nineteen a day for a week and so on until you're down to five a day. Once you're down to five a day you should be able to kick the habit completely.

If you see someone smoking, imagine what it's doing to their lungs, imagine the harm they are breathing into their bodies, and imagine how disgusting they will smell. For anyone that doesn't smoke, it is a total turn-off. Your breath smells stale and rank, your clothes smell, your fingers are stained with nicotine, and your fitness (performance) levels are way down. That horrible smoker's cough in the morning is not really what anyone wants to wake up next to either. And certainly not what anyone wants to kiss. In other words, the very opposite of sexy.

Be selfish—think about how much better you're going to feel and look. Smoking is the single most aging thing you can do to your body. Just think about all those women with wrinkles all around their lips, looking years

Spend the time you would have spent smoking getting fit with IDEA 11, *Fitting in fitness.*

Try another idea...

older than they really are. Also imagine the money you will save. It's an old tip, but a good idea is to put aside the money you would have spent on cigarettes and spend it on something special like a facial or a meal out every week. Or save up for a month and take your loved one away for a dirty weekend. A much more sensible way to spend your money.

There are lots of websites designed to help you in your struggle as well. For example, they give advice on how to cope with fidgety hands as well as providing encouraging statistics. If you want to buy your quit smoking products online then go to one of several sites selling products, but shop around, as prices vary. They sell all sorts of goodies from lozenges to nasal sprays. If you feel you need a little extra motivation then try some hypnotherapy CDs; there are lots of them in stores and online.

"A cigarette is the perfect type of pleasure. It is exquisite, and it leaves one unsatisfied."
OSCAR WILDE

Defining idea...

How did it go?

Q **I think about cigarettes all the time. What can I do?**

A *Look at it this way: It's either the cigarettes or you. You only have one go at life and this thing could very easily kill you. How stupid is that? Is it really worth it? I remember once walking through a cancer ward in a hospital in Italy. There was a man dying from lung cancer in one of the beds screaming, "Get the ceiling off me, it's collapsed on my chest." Whenever I thought about having a cigarette, I thought about him. Give it some time and you'll start to feel so much better. And your sex appeal rating will go up, too.*

Q **My boyfriend smokes. I used to find it attractive but now I just hate it. What can I do to get him to give it up?**

A *Treat him like you would a naughty child. Reward and reprimand. If he smokes, refuse to kiss him. If he manages a day without cigarettes, then reward him with a sexy treat. Very simple and most effective.*

14

Sensuous surroundings

The chaise longue—what a piece of furniture. It immediately conjures up images of sordid seventeenth-century sex. Take a look at the film _Dangerous Liaisons_ with Glenn Close and John Malkovich if you don't know what I'm talking about.

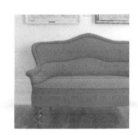

Sex on a bed is great, but don't ignore the potential of other pieces of furniture for creating a sexy mood and acting as great props.

If you're getting bored with sex in bed think about how to use your home to its best potential. And try to think of your furnishings not just as practical objects but things that enhance the way you feel when you walk into a room, sort of like a new dress makes you feel when you wear it. Surround yourself with beautiful and sensuous objects.

But while we're on the subject of beds—there are beds and there are beds. In terms of sexy beds, the one to have has got to be the four-poster. It conjures up images of long afternoons spent in bed, white sheets rustling, and bondage. It is a unique piece

Here's an idea for you... **Explore every room in your home for new sexy possibilities and think how a simple prop may transform a room into a sex den. Invest in a sheepskin rug for in front of your fireplace and suddenly you're transported to your own romantic log cabin. A dozen candles to light your bathroom will turn it into a sensual spa. The possibilities are endless.**

of furniture in that it can combine the romantic with the pervy. Nowadays you don't even have to pay a fortune for one. Lots of department stores have them and look online as well.

The chaise longue and four-poster are two classic pieces of sexy furniture, but for the more adventurous of you there are modern classics like the Sexy Lips Sofa. This is based on an original 1938 design called the Mae West Lips Sofa, created by Salvador Dali and Edward Jones. It is the ultimate in sexy kitsch and a must-have for a bachelor pad. To go along with it you can also buy the lipstick lamp (extremely phallic).

But don't ignore what you already have. There are ways to make your seemingly innocent furniture take on a whole new sexy glow. The first is to think of them as props for sex. OK, so if you're really dedicated you can buy all sorts of weird things like the inflatable bondage chair or a love swing (you suspend it from the ceiling and get into strange positions on it, but what do you say when your in-laws visit and ask you why there's a hole in the ceiling?) but improvising is just as much fun. Who can forget the brilliant sex scene with Jessica Lange and Jack Nicholson in *The Postman Always Rings Twice*? And what were they having sex on? A good old kitchen table. No inflatable bondage chairs for Jack. He just threw her on the table, flour going everywhere, and fulfilled the fantasy of many bored housewives.

Lighting is hugely important, too. Don't forget that to create the right atmosphere you need just the right amount of light. I'm sure you'll agree there's nothing more off-putting than walking into a restaurant ready for an intimate dinner and finding the place lit with neon lights. Invest in lamps with dimmer switches or table lamps or stand alone lamps as an alternative to the ceiling light. There are plenty of affordable, chic examples.

Enjoy a sexy evening in and take advantage of your sexy furniture. See IDEA 23, *There's no place like home.*

Try another idea...

Smell also plays a big part in the way a room feels. Invest in some fabulous products to make your home smell sweet and clean. Candles, incense, sprays, and essential oils can all add a sensual aroma, but be sure to go for the more classy and subtle ones rather than a cheap air freshener. Scented candles are lovely as they also create wonderful light.

"Home is where the heart is."
LATE 19TH-CENTURY PROVERB

Defining idea...

How did it go?

Q **I feel a little strange climbing all over the furniture to have sex. I mean, really, is this a good idea?**

A *Of course it is. But you shouldn't act like you've been planning it all day. Just grab the moment and don't think too deeply about it. You could pounce on your loved one in the bathroom for example and take things from there. Or tell him/her you've been thinking about having sex on a particular chair all day (in fact, chairs are great—he sits, she straddles). All you need to do is use your imagination. Think laterally.*

Q **Are you really suggesting I buy furniture in order to have sex on it?**

A *No, but you should buy furniture that is attractive and makes you feel good, not just the first table or chair you come across. Create a sexy environment in your home and the rest will follow.*

15

Sexy style

Image, style, look. Call it what you want, but you need to define it. Your style is something that is all about you.

You can change things, add accessories, lose weight, put on more lipstick, but unless you ooze your own personal style, it won't make much difference to your sex appeal.

A friend of mine was recently extremely irritated with her husband. They have been married for five years and he won't let her wear her old leggings around the house. "I know they're not the most attractive item of clothing I have," she says, "but they're so comfortable and I love them. He says they look awful and he doesn't want to see me in them." Some of you might say that's unreasonable, but I have begun to side with the husband in this argument. My friend would never have worn her old leggings on their first date. So why lose your sexy style just because you're married? Surely being married is even more reason to make an effort, unless you want your husband to start looking for sexy, stylish women elsewhere. Sexy style is something that should stay with you forever, your own intangible look and image; leggings are for those rare moments alone or with other girlfriends who also have comfort clothing they're longing to wear.

Here's an idea for you...

Transparent blouses are wonderfully sexy and no matter how little you like the idea there's a way to wear see-through without showing a thing. Fabric technology allows wispy fabrics to give just a hazy idea of what might be underneath. But if that's still too much, wear a jacket over it so there's only a glimpse of what's underneath. Also, a glimpse of lace works wonders.

So what style will you go for today? There are three classic looks that work well—romantic (flowing skirts), flirtatious (tight, short), and erotic (gorgeous clinging fabrics, seriously grown up). Obviously the image you choose is determined by where you are going and what you're going to be doing. It would be crazy to show up for a walk on the beach with your latest paramour wearing a leather skirt and stilettos. If it's a simple style you're after, try a pretty floral dress (or jeans if you're a guy), chinos and T-shirt, a flowing skirt and a cashmere sweater, and go for soft colors such as beige, light blue, or rose.

For a first date where there will be plenty of flirting going on, dress accordingly; a low-cut top or a short skirt (but never both together). Go for warm, passionate colors like red, and remember your choice of underwear is crucial.

The vampy, flirtatious look is really not the one for a first date. You could come across as cheap and tarty, which he might think is ideal for that night but won't be any good for your long-term prospects. Unless, of course, you're just after a hugely erotic one-night stand, in which case, go for it. If you do want to dress in a way that guarantees he'll want to sleep with you then, of course, leather is good (preferably black). Animal prints are also pretty effective as is anything seriously short and figure hugging. Lots of cleavage (if you don't have it, fake it), zips in strategic places, and lace-up tops are also safe bets.

Remember, you are in control of the image you want to portray and the signals you want to send out to your date. Don't make them the wrong ones by either going over the top or showing up looking like an elderly aunt, though some men may get off even on that look. Best not to risk it though.

You can relax stylishly, too. For more on that go to IDEA 19, Yes, we have no pajamas.

Try another idea...

"Penguins mate for life. Which doesn't exactly surprise me that much 'cause they all look alike—it's not like they're gonna meet a better looking penguin some day."
ELLEN DEGENERES, comedian

Defining idea...

How did it go?

Q **Are you saying I need to look hot the whole time? How about just relaxing for a change?**

A *Of course you can relax, but do it stylishly. There's nothing uncomfortable about a cashmere sweater or a chic T-shirt and pair of jeans. There is even some rather sexy and stylish housewear clothing around these days, which is a great alternative to jammies or sweatpants.*

Q **What about makeup?**

A *Makeup is crucial. Your makeup should reflect your clothes. Do not mix a summery pink cashmere top and flowing skirt with the red lips look. Instead, go for a little pale lip gloss. The little black dress can look great with thick, black eyelashes and red lips. Obviously, makeup depends very much on your complexion and coloring. Get professional advice if you're not sure. Any department store cosmetics counter will help. Don't forget that scent is important, and try to match your fragrance to your image. Some classics go with anything, but you don't want to send out contradicting messages, so take care.*

16

Musical mystique

Since time began music has been a great aphrodisiac. In _Don Giovanni_ the great man seduces his victim with a compelling aria, and Marvin Gaye has had us all writhing around to "Sexual Healing."

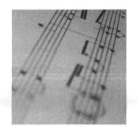

Everybody has a song that brings back special memories and it's often the one you first kissed to or fell in love to.

When you're feeling less than sexy, music is your greatest ally in getting you in the mood for love. Music can enhance or change your feelings in a heartbeat. And the memory of an ultra-sexy moment to music will stay with you forever; the musical memory is very powerful. The importance of music in sex cannot be exaggerated. It can change a whole mood. It can wreck or make a situation. Whether you find classical or popular music turns you on, it's the easiest way of taking you from not interested to raring to go.

So, you're ready for that all-important date. This is the night. It's dinner at your place. What music do you choose to set the mood? I like classical music, but as I know this isn't everyone's choice, I will keep it brief. The most seductive piece of

Here's an idea for you… **If you're having a seductive dinner with your loved one, try something classical. It's wise to steer clear of opera as it can get a bit screechy and spoil an intimate moment. Try soul for raunchy sex and Brazilian samba when you want to get really hot and passionate. Something mellow and atmospheric works well for the aperitif. Just make sure it's not going to make you sleepy.**

operatic music for me is the aria from *Don Giovanni*, where he seduces Elvira. It has a flow and a pace that just makes you want to fall into bed with the Don yourself. He tells her to give him her hand and explains how she will say yes. She protests that she feels sorry for her fiancé. The Don tells her he will change her life. But be careful—if you end up smooching to this you might get a rude awakening when the earth opens and Hell claims the evil seducer at the end, rather loudly. A more relaxing option might be Mozart's Clarinet Concerto, my all-time favorite piece of music. I first heard it on a Walkman lying by a pool on one of my first ever trips abroad with my husband. It seemed to me the most perfect piece of music ever written: flowing, seductive, entrancing. Just listen to it and tell me it doesn't move you. You might recognize it as the tune Robert Redford and Meryl Streep danced to on her terrace in *Out of Africa*.

You could always invite your partner to dance, not necessarily to Mozart, but how about some slow and sexy blues music? Don't be self-conscious about it, just dim the lights, move the furniture out of the way, put on your favorite tune, and go for it. Better still, strip to something seductive. This might sound unlikely but I have a very good friend who once did a strip to Schubert's *Ave Maria* in front of her lover in a hotel room in Prague. If you don't know it, go and listen to it immediately. It has a wonderful build-up and the mixture between soothing, seductive, and dramatic is perfect to strip to. Probably not what the composer intended when he wrote his tribute to the Virgin Mary! If you're unsure of how to strip then take some tips from the professionals. There are lots of films about strippers such as Demi Moore's *Striptease,* or take a tip from the French. The biggest department store there hired girls from the Crazy Horse club to show customers how to remove underwear seductively. Rent *Moulin Rouge* and get some tips from Nicole Kidman.

If you're able to, seduce your partner with some music of your own. My in-laws knew a man who used to serenade his wife up to bed every night from a grand piano at the bottom of the stairs. The couple in question are sadly no longer with us but I like to think he is still serenading her somewhere up there. It's never too late to learn to play the piano and there's nothing guaranteed to gain you more kudos than the ability to swing insouciantly onto a piano stool and give your loved one a tune.

Make your own music—learn to play a musical instrument in IDEA 20, *Play away.*

Try another idea...

"If music be the food of love, play on."
WILLIAM SHAKESPEARE, *Twelfth Night*

Defining idea...

69

Q **The person I am trying to seduce is a music lover. How can I impress her?**

A *Take her to the opera on a first date. Remember Richard Gere and Julia Roberts in* Pretty Woman*? He takes her to see* La Traviata *and she is totally overwhelmed. Opera is a great aphrodisiac when done well. I remember standing through a whole performance of* Eugene Onegin *once and falling desperately in love with my date, even though he couldn't afford seats.*

Q **I find it too embarrassing to strip. I get all self-conscious. What can I do to loosen my inhibitions?**

A *Yes, so do we all, except possibly the professionals. First tip, drink something beforehand. But not too much; there's nothing as ungainly as a drunk stripper falling over her stilettos as she tries to ease off a stocking. Second tip, dim the lights. In fact, turn them off and go for candles instead. Final tip, relax and let yourself be seduced by the whole mood and music as well. Remember that the key to being sexy is confidence. You know you can do it. Get in touch with your inner tramp.*

17

Flirt, flirt, flirt

There is nothing, and I mean nothing, quite as sexy as someone who knows how to flirt correctly. They can make your toes tingle and your legs turn to jelly.

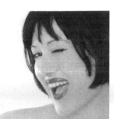

Amazingly, when you first meet someone, the initial impression you make on them will depend 55 percent on your appearance and body language, 38 percent on your style of speaking, and only 7 percent on what you actually say.

Flirting or conveying that you like someone depends on all sorts of things that are not linked to speech. The most important factor is eyes. Think about how long you maintain eye contact with people. Usually we limit eye contact to brief glances. This is because actually looking someone in the eye for any length of time is an indicator of intense emotion. In fact, it is usually either an act of love, lust, or hate. Use this reluctance to maintain eye contact to your own advantage. You can show your interest in someone simply by making eye contact across the room and holding their gaze for a split-second more than you normally would. (Don't do much more or you might end up looking like a crazed lunatic.) If your "victim" maintains eye

Here's an idea for you... **When you smile, try to project the feeling of "I'm so happy to be here talking to you" in a totally natural way, of course. Someone who seems to take genuine delight in your presence is almost impossible to resist.**

contact, then chances are he or she feels the same way and your paths will meet in the not-so-distant future. Initial eye contact combined with an eyebrow flash (raising the eyebrow very briefly) can be deadly. Obviously, if you've had Botox during the past month this won't be an option (don't risk it, your eyebrow might get stuck up there).

Once your gazes meet, you need to start thinking about other things as well as the all-important eyes. The distance you put between you, for instance. In continental Europe the so-called "personal zone" is smaller than in the US, so if you're talking to a Spanish girl and she's really close to you, you shouldn't assume she is flirting. This might just be a manifestation of a cultural difference and not lust. However, in the US any closer than two small steps away and you're in the flirt zone. If you are not sure you're wanted, try moving a little closer and watching the reaction of your intended. If she keels back and crosses her arms in front of her then you can assume she's either chronically shy or not interested. Crossed legs are another sign that you're not on to a winner, as is rubbing the back of the neck. If the object of your desire leans toward you or starts echoing your posture (i.e., copying what you do) then things are looking good.

Obviously, all these signs you are looking out for are also things you can be doing in order to signal your interest in the other person. Another thing you should do (and will be doing if you're interested in sleeping with this person) is to act animated. Use gestures and be lively and interested in what they have to say: Men love nothing more than a girl hanging on their every word. Women should be careful not to let the initial interest shown by a man encourage them to relate their life story. He may act like it's the most riveting thing since the World Series, but trust me, it's not.

Now that you know how to flirt, find out how to be good in bed. See IDEA 41, *Sexy sex*.

Try another idea...

When things start to heat up you can try a little touch. I'm not talking a lunge for the breasts, guys, but a light and fleeting brush with your hand across her forearm. If used appropriately, touch can move things forward very fast, but you need to be careful. A touch too soon can ruin the atmosphere and have your intended one running for cover. Finally, think about your verbal flirtation skills. What you say (obviously) is important, but so is the tone of your voice. The simple and short word "hello" can have different connotations depending on how it is pronounced. It can convey that you are bored or that you are delighted. Remember that when it comes to first impressions, your style of speaking has far greater influence on people's reactions than what you say.

"Merely innocent flirtation, not quite adultery, but adulteration."
LORD BYRON

Defining idea...

How did it go?

Q   I'm terrible at flirting. What can I do?

A   *Get out there and practice with anyone moderately attractive that you meet, not just someone you are interested in. Practice on the store clerk, waiter, ticket collector. The more you do it, the better you'll get and your confidence will grow every day. And above all, see what works and what doesn't. Learn from trial and error.*

Q   Is it OK to flirt with other people's spouses?

A   *Yes, of course. That's partly what they're there for. As Byron says, it is not adultery. Flirting makes us feel attractive, young, and confident if it is reciprocated. Go for it, but just be careful not to overstep the boundaries. You might end up with a very grumpy spouse, and that's just your own.*

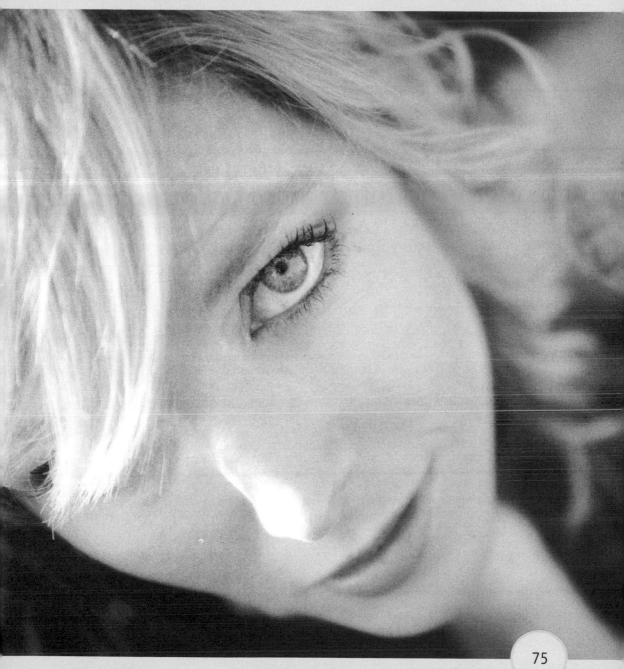

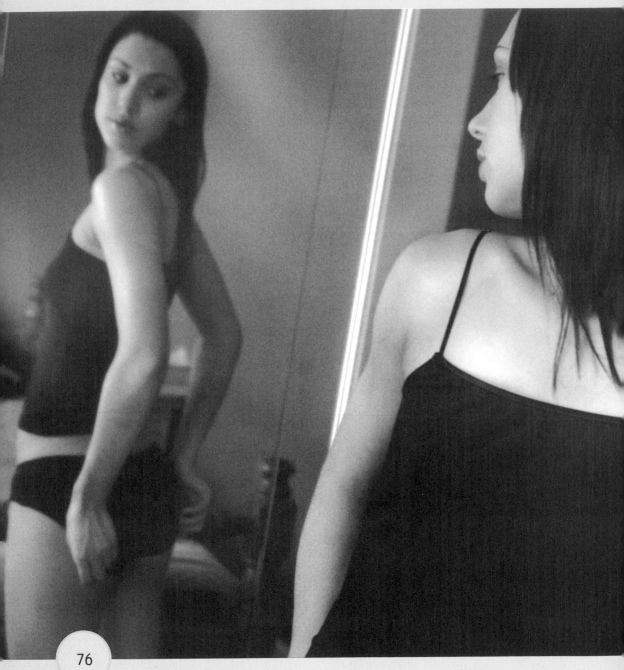

18

Tricks of the trade

It's finally happened: The date you have been waiting for for six months is on. The man of your dreams is going to meet you, just you, for a totally romantic time and it's going to happen . . . tonight.

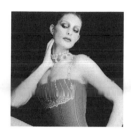

Help! You still can't get into those jeans you swore you would diet your way into a year ago. Your waistline is way over its ideal and you have three hours to change it.

No point in dieting now. Reach for those panties of steel. Remember Bridget Jones? These miracle workers basically compress your flesh and reduce your waistline. You can get those that reach down to your thighs as well. They come in all shapes and sizes with reassuring names like "body slimmers" and "hi-waist busters." They can be found on the Web and in department stores. "Quite miraculously, these can—and do—take a couple of inches off your waist and stop you from looking like you're four months pregnant," says India Knight in her book *The Shops*, "without the excess flesh making a reappearance elsewhere."

Here's an idea for you... **The cosmetics counter can also help. Fake tan, firming and lifting serums, and exfoliators can all make a contribution. Try those that offer an instant toning effect. Rub them on any skin that is on show and watch it glow.**

Another, less restricting option is tights. Lots of retailers sell ranges of slimming tights, which are great but take forever to peel off due to their compressing nature. (Panties of steel are not easy to take off either; you'll need a very determined date to get around them. In short, this is underwear to wear to impress as opposed to seduce.)

One thing that can be both slimming and seductive is a corset. I once had a Vivienne Westwood corset that had the most amazing effect on my (nonexistent) chest. As a result, I felt incredibly sexy wearing it. It was also very slimming on the waist, although when I last tried it on (three children and fifteen years later) the waist was a bit too high to be really flattering, so it's now in the dressing-up box. I have now moved on to Paris-based Chantal Thomass's corsets. My particular favorite is leopard skin (what midlife crisis?). Her products are available in large department stores and other lingerie outlets worldwide. A corset will set you back around $200, but it's worth it purely for the effect it has on your waist and breasts. Wear it with jeans and a cashmere cardigan to achieve the greatest sexy impact.

Don't forget the top half, too. Minimizing bras can contribute to a svelte shape. This is not a garment I have ever had to wear but I gather from a friend who has that problem is one of excess flesh squashed down by the bra turning up in strange places. My advice would be to ditch the minimizing bra and strut your chest with pride. Men love boobs, there's no denying it. For those of you with little or no chest (like me), there is the maximizing bra or Wonderbra. This is an essential piece of clothing. It is worth spending proper money on this, as cheap ones are rarely as effective.

Sexiness is all about confidence and these little props will help you feel gorgeous and boost your ego.

If you've got more time to get fit, then go for IDEA 25, Sporting chance.

Try another idea...

"Love is just a system for getting someone to call you darling after sex."
JULIAN BARNES

Defining idea...

79

How did it go?

Q   What is the point of wearing panties of steel when he's going to see what you really look like when he gets them off?

A   *Fair point, but the image of you waltzing into the room looking serene and thin will stay with him forever. Image is everything in the seduction game. The better you feel about the way you look the more you are going to ooze confidence and sexiness. I promise you it's worth a try. Those panties of steel really do work wonders and, miraculously, one can still breathe while wearing them. When it comes to undressing, dim the lights. In fact, turn them off!*

Q   How about not eating anything at all the day of the date? Surely then I'll look thinner?

A   *Possibly, but you might also get horribly drunk and light-headed and fall over on your way to the restroom. Not a good look. By all means, don't stuff your face, eat in moderation, and do not eat any garlic under any circumstances. Also be aware of foods that make you bloated (possibly some fruits and vegetables) and avoid them. Huge amounts of fizzy water will bloat you, too. Avoiding fizzy drinks is an obvious tip, but that goes for all the time, not just before a date. Another thing to avoid is chewing gum, which can make you feel bloated. Ideally, eat something light like some lean meat or chicken before heading out to keep you from being ravenous but that avoids enlarging your silhouette.*

19

Yes, we have no pajamas

It's cold outside. In fact, it's cold inside. All you really want to do is to get into your full-length flannel nightie and snuggle up in bed.

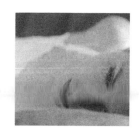

But you can't—not if you want to be sexy.

When asked what she wore in bed, Marilyn Monroe replied, "Chanel No. 5." I'm not suggesting you wear nothing in the middle of winter, but there are ways to avoid looking like a furry toy. The key is silk. There is nothing more comfortable and warm than a pair of silk pajamas. OK, so there's probably not much that's more expensive either, but a good pair should last you forever and you can go to bed knowing you look great and will be snug as a bug. While we're on the subject of splurging on nightwear, a friend of mine once shocked the hell out of me by spending over $500 on a cashmere dressing gown from Ralph Lauren. I thought she'd gone totally bonkers. For $500 you could fly to the Caribbean. "You could," she said, "but my dressing gown will be with me forever." Fifteen years later, she's still got it and it looks great. Light, flowing, soft but oh-so-cozily warm. Total heaven. Working it out, she's paid less than $40 a year to own this item—I now wish I'd bought one, too.

Here's an idea for you...

When you are sleeping alone (not often, obviously, you sex-goddess), treat your hands and feet to a serious moisturizing treatment. Put thick cream or oil on your feet and hands and massage well. This should be done once you're in bed so you don't kill yourself skidding over the floor to get there. Another good tip (strictly for when you're alone) is to put on a moisturizing face pack and leave it on all night, and try to get to bed early. It's thought that an hour before midnight is worth two after.

Nightwear is a great thing to think about. It conjures up all sorts of sexy images. It is perhaps hard to believe but the sort of thing you wear at night can define your image. If you go to bed dressed like a playboy bunny, chances are you'll get treated like one. Now that even department stores sell sexy nightwear there is no longer any excuse for you to get into bed looking like a grandmother. It's fine working hard all day long to look sexy, but it's essential to keep up that image at nighttime, too. This applies even if you are sleeping alone—it'll help reinforce your self-image as a sensual creature. Don't just give up and put on your grey (were once white) cotton underwear. Think creatively, sexily, and come up with something a little different. You can buy all sorts of cute little night outfits. Short nighties, for example, simple cuts with perhaps a ribbon or two, even if they're made of cotton, are a good choice. Please go for good quality, though—polyester and other man-made fibers don't allow your skin to breathe, and while sweating is fine in bed, it should be from exertion, not from simply overheating. Go for natural fibers such as cotton and silk, whatever design you choose. The one exception to this is when you're going for the Playboy look, in which case it needs to be red, glossy, and totally fake—you probably won't end up keeping it on for long anyway.

I like those little panty and top ensembles. They can be very simple and really cute— understatedly sexy, especially if they're made from cotton. They don't make you look like you're making a huge effort to look sexy, but are slightly different and popular with men.

Get ready for an early night with a relaxing, sexy bath. See **IDEA 24,** *The art of the sexy bath.*

Try another idea...

You can also, of course, go for the Marilyn Monroe recipe and wear nothing but your favorite scent in bed. For this look, you need to be smooth, soft, and gorgeously clean or the effect will be lost. So wax, shave, whatever it is you do to stay stubble-free, then shower or bathe. An added bonus for soft skin is to exfoliate beforehand, preferably with exfoliating gloves. In fact, if you do this three times a week you'll be amazed at the difference it makes. After exfoliating, smother yourself with gorgeous smelling moisturizing lotion or body oil. Similarly, don't overdo the scent, as there aren't many other smells in bed to detract from it. Try this trick: Spray a cloud of it just in front of you and walk through it. You should come out the other end smelling just sweet enough.

"As you make your bed, so you must lie upon it."
LATE 15TH-CENTURY FRENCH PROVERB

Defining idea...

How did it go?

Q **Surely there's no point to all of this. It's dark at night anyway.**

A *Wrong. Of course there is a point. Your image is all-important, whatever the time of day or night. If you feel gorgeous you'll be more confident day and night. And anyway, by the morning it will be light.*

Q **Some of this stuff is really expensive. Isn't it a waste to wear it at night?**

A *Don't think of it as just wearing it at night. We spend a quarter of our lives asleep, and probably more in bed. These hours take up a great chunk of your life and you need to be properly dressed. Obviously in order to be properly undressed.*

20

Play away

There was a reason that playing the piano well used to be essential in attracting a good husband.

You look terrific playing an instrument and those who do it well send out the message that they are sensitive and passionate— qualities that transfer well to the bedroom and are endlessly sexy.

Things have changed, but that's no reason to ignore the power of music. I went to a lunch party recently with some friends. They have teenage daughters, all of whom were, as you might expect, ignoring us. Until one of the men in our group started playing the electric guitar (he never travels without it). Suddenly, one teenage daughter got her drum kit out, the other started strumming her electric guitar, and both of them were gazing in awe at my friend, who is an extremely good musician. "I'm a chick magnet," he grinned as *Wonderwall* flowed effortlessly from his fingers. This is possibly true. But only because they were attracted by his ability to produce music.

Here's an idea for you...

If you're not interested in going to classes, then try to learn online. There are lots of websites that offer lessons for free as a starter. Make the first tune you try to learn one of your favorites. Just hearing the first few bars will inspire you to keep going. It's amazing how quickly you will make progress.

Music is something that almost everyone likes. So playing a musical instrument is not like being able to hang glide, which is likely to make you popular with only a limited number of people. You can entertain, seduce, impress, amuse, and titillate people with a tune. Being musical is something that attracts people and is a really positive accomplishment to cultivate. It can also be incredibly sexy. I have seen grown men practically swoon at the sight of Jacqueline du Pré with her cello between her legs. The passion and the power she gave out was incredible and inspiring. She was a beautiful lady as well, but think about Luciano Pavarotti, whose voice can almost be defined as an instrument in itself. The man is so obese he can barely move and yet he is still undeniably a babe magnet.

So what can you do if you don't play a musical instrument or you're tone deaf? Focus on your other assets? No, not at all. The friend I mentioned earlier started playing the guitar in his thirties. He managed to teach himself and now he plays as if he's been doing it all his life. Learning a musical instrument is possible at any age. And like any talent or accomplishment, it makes you more attractive. I started to learn to play the piano when I was thirty and progressed faster than I could have imagined. It was such a buzz to play my first ever piece of music. With music, there is no downside, only good can come of learning to play an instrument. It's fun, rewarding, and challenging.

The type of music you want to play will help you decide what musical instrument to go for; if you want versatility then go for the guitar or piano. Remember, too, that it is harder to get a decent note out of some instruments than others, so if you want to feel like you are progressing quickly and be able to play tunes right away, it's probably best to steer clear of the violin, trombone, or bagpipes.

If you can't yet play a musical instrument, then dance the night away. Turn to IDEA 4, *Dance yourself sexy*.

Try another idea...

Musical instruments can be expensive, so don't invest in a grand piano or harp unless you're absolutely certain. If you want to try out a musical instrument to see how you progress many music shops will rent instruments (often new ones) out to you and may include an option where the instrument is yours after a certain number of monthly payments. As a guide, you can expect monthly prices to start at the equivalent of a couple of good bottles of wine for a smaller instrument such as a flute. Once you want to buy an instrument then shopping online can get you some very competitive prices.

If you want to take lessons then you can expect to pay the equivalent of your two bottles of wine again for half an hour of tuition. Students studying music at a university will often teach music in their spare time—like all other students they are short of cash—and they may offer lower prices than professional musicians (or perhaps just take the wine).

"Music and women I cannot but give way to, whatever my business is."
SAMUEL PEPYS

Defining idea...

Once you have progressed a little then why not join a band, orchestra, or other local music group? That way you can meet other like-minded and sexy individuals—who knows where it'll lead?

How did
it go?

Q   **I just don't think I can face it. Isn't it like trying to learn another language?**

A   *Yes, it is, as Barry White would say, the language of love . . . but there's no doubt it's worth it. Just give it a try. Book ten lessons for the instrument of your choice and see them out. You might find you have hidden talents.*

Q   **Surely I will just look and sound like an amateur for the rest of my life.**

A   *It all depends on how much time and effort you're prepared to spend. As I said, a friend of mine started to play the guitar in his thirties and now plays effortlessly. It's probably not a good idea to go straight for something complicated like the cello, so choose something a little easier to handle. The guitar or banjo are ideal. Don't laugh—the banjo played well is a real turn-on. I promise!*

21

Feed your desires

Cooking is the new sex. New and exciting celebrity chefs have seen to that. They are masters of tasting, cooking, preparing, chopping, and frying, and they do it with such flair that we're glued to the screen.

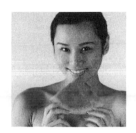

So how do you harness some of that seductive cooking style for yourself?

Cooking is a no-brainer when it comes to seduction. Women love to be cooked for—it makes them feel protected and cared for. And the way to a man's heart really is through his stomach. No, really. New research into the sort of foods that make each sex happiest showed that while women enjoy snacks (no cooking involved), men like proper meals. They associate them with being loved. So cook up a storm for your lover and you can't go wrong.

As a sexy hostess you can't be stressed. So the key is in the preparation. Do as much as you can the day before. Some things, like a tiramisu pudding, for example, actually need to be prepared the day before, as they taste much better if they can sit for a night. When you are planning what to serve keep an eye out for dishes that can be prepared the day before and just reheated (or defrosted) before you eat.

Here's an idea for you...

There's no need to complicate things. What would be sexier than high quality vanilla ice cream with hot chocolate sauce poured over it? It is the easiest thing in the world to make. Just break some luxury dark chocolate into a bowl (make sure it is at least 70 percent cocoa solids), place the bowl over a saucepan of boiling water, turn the heat down, and let it slowly melt. If it looks a little too thick then add some cream just before taking it off the heat, adding a few roasted flaked almonds as a finishing touch. Three aphrodisiacs in one dish. Perfect.

So what to feed them? How do you define sexy food? Sexy food is food that tastes and looks good and that requires a certain amount of handling. Crudités with dips, for example, can be made sexy. They are healthy, tasty, and can be eaten very seductively. Try to stick to carrots, cucumber, zucchini, and radishes. Broccoli and cauliflower can give people gas, which is not good for the party atmosphere and very far from sensual.

What you cook will, of course, depend on the season and where you live. When available, oysters are an obvious choice since they are supposedly an aphrodisiac and perceived as very sexy. They have practically no calories, are full of protein, and are very high in zinc, which is said to enhance male fertility, potency, and sex drive since it is essential to sperm production. A single oyster contains a man's daily requirement of zinc. Chocolate contains an ingredient that apparently increases the blood flow to the genitals, and the chemicals in cocoa solids increase sexual desire. A rather more surprising aphrodisiac is celery, which contains androsterone, the male hormone. Research suggests that if men eat celery, they sweat andosterone and thus attract women; some say celery also stimulates the gland in the brain that controls sex hormones. Ginseng, cloves, grapes, fennel, almonds, bananas, walnuts, ginger, chili, chickpeas, vanilla, berries (strawberries, blackberries, and raspberries are packed with vitamins C and E, which increase your sex drive), and asparagus are all desire stimulants, too.

Now that you've mastered the art of sexy cooking, try sexy drinking. IDEA 51, *Bottoms up*, will give you some tips on this.

Try another idea...

There are lots of diet plans packed with high aphrodisiac foods. These are based on the idea that eating things that are full of nutrients your body needs to cope with stress, tiredness, and hormonal swings (which can all lower your libido) will have you ready for action. Try a healthy eating plan for at least seven days, increasing your water intake and cutting out alcohol or at least reducing the quantity you consume. Include lots of fruits and vegetables, especially berries, which you can eat with yogurt and flaked almonds. Other high sex appeal items include salad niçoise; asparagus; feta cheese and basil omelette; spicy grilled shrimp; chicken breasts baked with cherry tomatoes, basil, and garlic; salmon fillets with ginger and pine nuts; oatcakes with hummus; and plain chocolate. Whatever else you achieve you'll find that you'll be constantly thinking about sex and feel like it more often. I'm going to try cooking exclusively from the aphrodisiac food list at my next dinner party and see what happens.

"It is good food and not fine words that keeps me alive."
MOLIÈRE

Defining idea...

91

Q   How can I look serene and sexy with a kitchen full of food and a mess everywhere?

A   The key to entertaining is preparation. Do as much as you can the day before and as much as you can on the day before anyone arrives. Don't waste too much valuable time meticulously cleaning your house; no one will notice. Also be sure to have at least an hour between all the preparation and the guests arriving to unwind, get showered, and prepare yourself.

Q   What about if it's just the two of us?

A   Then you can get really sexy. Think 9 ½ Weeks—in other words, food you can feed each other and enjoy. Good examples are strawberries with or without whipped cream; ice cream, preferably something really decadent with lots of naughty bits; melted marshmallows in front of an open fire; spaghetti eaten seductively opposite each other (elegantly please, and no spoons, ask any Italian).

22
Enduring allure

It's not difficult to feel sexy at the beginning of a relationship. That first kiss is one of the most memorable things ever. Just the touch of your lover's hand will give you goose bumps.

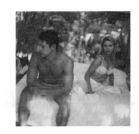

But that sort of intensity doesn't last forever. Sadly, it goes with time and with familiarity. What can you do to rekindle it?

I once read a story about a couple who had been together for years and got bored with one another. One night they both went to a party. For some reason, she ended up naked in the host's bedroom. The lights were out, her husband came in and got into bed with her. They had fabulous sex and each only realized afterward that they had slept with their spouse. Slightly far-fetched, but what it highlights is the fact that great sex needn't stop. It's all in the mind. These people hadn't had sex with each other for months. Because each thought he or she was with someone else, that it was forbidden, they had a great time.

Here's an idea for you...

One evening sit down and reminisce. Go through your first date, what you wore, what you did, the first time you had sex. Talk about all the things that first attracted you to each other. Was it the way he talked, something he said? Was it a certain skirt she wore, the way she flicked her hair? This should bring back happy memories and rekindle lustful thoughts.

So, you need to get the fact that you are an old boring married couple out of your mind and start thinking about all the things that drove you wild about each other. You are still the same people, if a little older and more familiar—you just need to rediscover each other.

If you are married or living with someone and have children, finding the time to rediscover each other is not always easy. If you possibly can, go away together alone at least once every three months or so. It's not just the fact of being alone that's important, it's being away from all the chores and worries of home. It's hard to feel sexy when all you can talk about is a burst pipe, ill children, and unpaid bills. You work all day, run the house, and collapse into bed exhausted at night. Not much time for sex. Try to think of sex as a priority and make time for it. Forget washing dishes, ironing, or watching hours of television in the evening. Slip into some sexy underwear and seduce your husband instead. What could be more important than that?

There are lots of little ways to make your everyday life sexier. Try to add spark to your life by thinking of each day as a day filled with sexy opportunities. Broaden your horizons. For example, don't just think of the bathroom as a place to shave, but a place to rekindle your romance.

For tips on spicing up your relationship, go to IDEA 39, *Spice up your life.*

Try another idea...

Being sexy is, of course, not just about looking good. Some friends of mine recently got divorced. The husband is a workaholic with his own business while the wife didn't work. "I just lost respect for her," he told me. "I couldn't bear to see her wasting time and achieving nothing. She seemed to have no ambition whatsoever, no respect for herself or her own status. In the end, she also had nothing to talk about, apart from what to eat or what the kids had done at school." He sounds harsh, but I see his point. He didn't care that his wife didn't work, but he did care that she never used her mind. There are those among us who want nothing more than the luxury of staying at home and raising our children, which is great as long as you don't forget that when you got married you were an interesting person in your own right and you need to ensure that you stay that way.

"Some people ask the secret of our long marriage. We take time to go to a restaurant two times a week. A little candlelit dinner, music, and dancing. She goes Tuesdays, I go Fridays."
HENNY YOUNGMAN, comedian

Defining idea...

How did it go?

Q **I just can't get interested in sex with my husband. It's simply the last thing I want to do. How can I remedy this?**

A *The first thing to do is not to beat yourself up about it. You may be tired, stressed, any number of things. But you can change how you feel. If it's a really desperate situation then go see a doctor, therapist, or alternative practitioner. Homeopathic doctors have medicines that help to heighten your libido. If you think it's something you can deal with yourself then you just have to get your head around it. Sometimes the thought of making the effort to have sex is worse than the actual action. Just get into it and let yourself go—it'll do you good.*

Q **Someone once told me we should make a date with each other. This seems ridiculous to me—we live together. Is it a crazy idea?**

A *No, believe me. Your lives are busy and the last thing you have time for is each other. Make a date and stick to it. It will make you feel special and do your relationship a lot of good. Decide to leave work early and meet for a drink on your way home, or meet for lunch or make a date to meet in the bath.*

23

There's no place like home

Couples should make an effort to go out with each other on dates. Otherwise, your partner becomes indistinguishable from the furniture and that's never going to be good for your sex life.

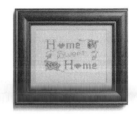

However, the exception is when you plan a date in your own home. A little effort on your part and you'll have the best cheap date of your life.

This idea works for all couples, but is especially sexy when you've been together for a while. If you have children, you want to get them out of the house for the evening before you start on the rest. Send the children to stay with their friends overnight (which they'll love) or with a willing relative or neighbor. Even if your kids are usually out like a light by 7:30, it is worthwhile to get complete privacy. Houses feel different without children in them, even if the children aren't visible, and you will feel less inhibited knowing you are completely alone.

What you do with this precious time is up to you, but I strongly advise transforming your home into a palace of love first. It's amazing how a little preparation can turn everyday surroundings into something very sexy. Most important is the lighting.

Here's an
idea for
you...

When you can't make a whole evening of it, you can at least go to bed early and lock the door. Make your bedroom as sensuous as possible. It's really worth investing in Egyptian cotton sheets, duvet covers, and pillowcases–they feel great and get softer the more you wash them. Strew rose petals on the bed, light the room with scented candles, draw the curtains, and relax. Don't forget to take the phone off the hook.

Absolutely no overhead or wall lights allowed. Throw some scarves over lamps or light at least a dozen candles for a lovely atmosphere (taking care at all times not to create a fire hazard). Put away all signs of family life— plastic toys, family pictures even—you don't want to be reminded of your mother mid-passionate embrace. Do everything you can to make your home sexy—get rid of clutter, briefcases, any reminder of work. Make sure the rooms are pleasantly warm.

Before you start make sure you have some sensuous food on hand—you might get hungry later. You can, of course, make the focus of the evening a romantic dinner à deux, but I'd advise against it. First, the food may well predominate, with one of you popping up to serve the next course; second, you might get a bit full and be ready for bed, but not in the right way. Instead, make sure you eat something in the early evening so you won't be starving and have some sexy food on hand like strawberries and whipped cream, artichokes and butter, ice cream—foods you can pick on, smear on each other, and generally get dirty with if the mood takes you.

Once the preparations are done, take turns getting ready for each other (a little separation at this point will build suspense). Make as much effort as if you were going out. Sip champagne while you get ready and think dirty thoughts.

Now for the real point of the evening—totally focusing on each other. Here are some ideas for starters.

For more tips on how to create a sexy haven at home, try IDEA 14, Sensuous surroundings.

Try another idea...

- If, as a couple, you need to reconnect, have a drink and a talk in front of the fire. This is not a chat about the gas bill or work prospects. You are allowed only to talk about your relationship and, to be safe, only the good things about your relationship. A good idea is to talk about your memories of when you met—first kiss, first date, first sex.

- Pretend you're strangers who have bumped into each other at a party. Sip drinks and get reacquainted all over again. Or make up a new alternative persona and pretend to be someone different, the kind of person you've always wanted to be. This is really good for letting your old partner see a new side of your personality, which can be very sexy.

- Decide to have sex in every room in your house.

- Play strip poker.

- Indulge in a bit of fantasy foreplay. Pick a couple of scenarios that appeal to you and act them out a little—strict boss and assistant, doctor and patient, plumber and frustrated housewife. A few props can help, as can a few drinks.

- Take a long bath or a steamy shower together.

Defining idea...

"Most of us find it all too easy to let life get in the way of love . . . If we can make any private time at all for each other, it's only when we're tired and distracted. [This means] the same old moves, the same old positions, and after a while sex gets boring."
LAURA CORN, bestselling sex book author

How did it go?

Q **We don't have any family nearby we can leave the kids with. Any suggestions?**

A. *Finding a sitter should be a priority assignment for you, although admittedly, it may take some time to find one since, clearly, you won't be happy leaving your kids with someone you don't trust 100 percent. If you have really good friends see if you can work out something. A good idea is to set up a babysitting swap rotation with another couple who, like you, want time together. One of you babysits for them one week, one of them babysits for you the next week. With time, it might be possible to organize sleepovers (for the children), although some couples won't go for it and it will depend on the individual children involved. But even if you never get to the stage of having the place to yourself for a whole night, at least you'll be getting free babysitting a few hours every few weeks—and that's got to be good.*

Q **Won't my wife think I'm cheap?**

A *If you are cheap, yes. If you are usually generous, no, she'll think you're being inventive. There's very little sexy about a cheap man, but to those of you who really think that romancing your missus is a waste of money, my advice is think quality not quantity. A $30 bouquet sent to her workplace out of the blue on a rainy Wednesday will be money very well spent. Showing that she's on your mind is very sexy—and doesn't have to cost a lot.*

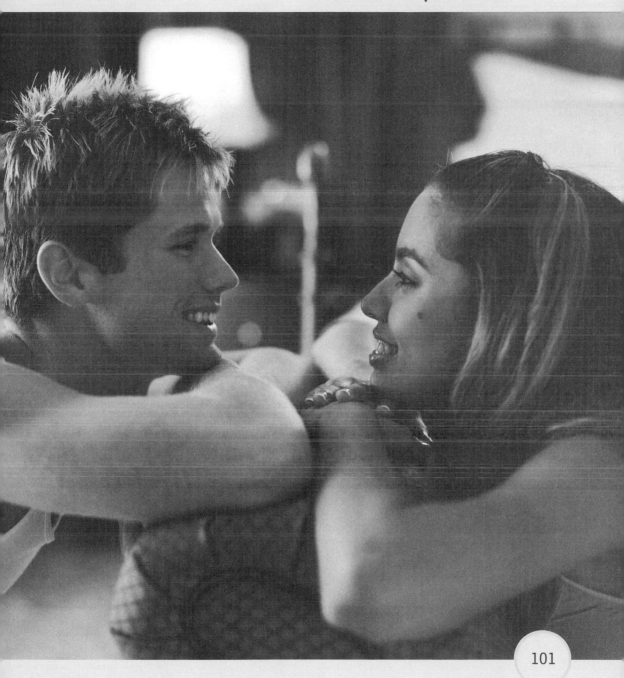

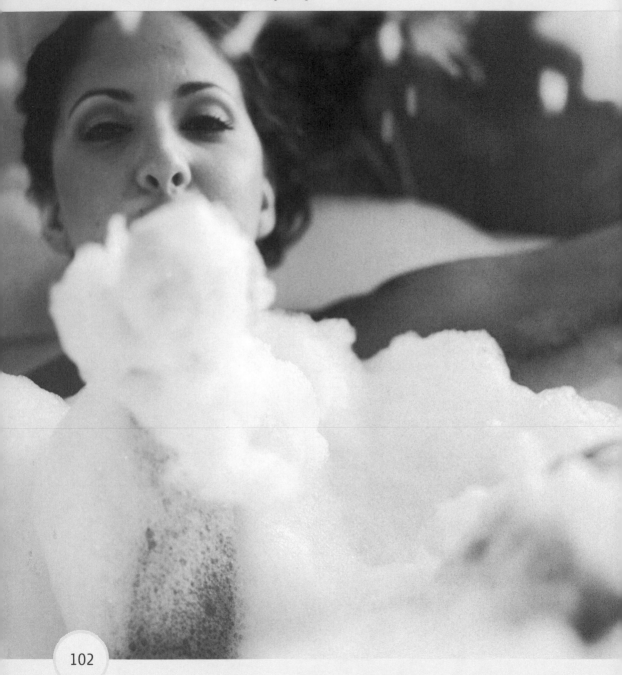

24

The art of the sexy bath

There is something unforgettable about your first bath with someone.

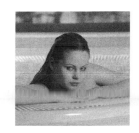

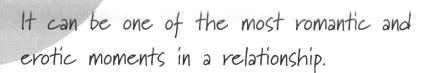
It can be one of the most romantic and erotic moments in a relationship.

Just taking a bath can make you feel better, and when your mood is lifted you'll be much more likely to feel sexy. The serenity, the calm, the scented candles. It's the one way to wash away all the day's troubles and regain your inner composure.

So how does one create that lovely, sexy atmosphere? Well, a large part is played by choosing the right lighting. Candles are the key—place them around the bath if there is room, or on the windowsill, or even put floating candles in the sink. You also need to get the temperature right; the water should be warm and inviting, the room cozy. There's nothing worse than getting out of a bath feeling like a shriveled lobster because it was too hot.

If you're after a gorgeous, relaxing bath just for yourself then here's what you do: While you're running the bath remove any makeup and nail polish. Then give yourself a dry body brush. This removes dead skin and stimulates circulation. Start at the soles of your feet and work upward, always brushing in the direction of the heart. Then wash your hair and put on an intensive treatment. Wrap a warmed-up

Here's an idea for you...

If you suffer from dry skin then try pouring a little baby oil into each bath. A little goes a long way, so don't overdo it or you'll be sliding around like a French fry in batter.

towel around your head or put your hair in a shower cap. Next, put on a face pack of your choice; moisturizing ones are especially good when you're relaxing.

Once you're ready, put the potions of your choice in the bath. When it comes to these, there are literally hundreds of products to choose from. Lots of foaming bath products will make you feel really glamorous, or you could try adding a small amount of essential oils of ylang-ylang or patchouli, both of which are said to have aphrodisiac properties. Mix a few drops of the oils with a little milk before adding them to the bath to ensure that they diffuse properly in the water. The whole room will smell great.

Put some mellow music on. Light your candles and turn the lights off. Sink into the bath, lean back, and relax. Once you've relaxed for about ten minutes it's time to start working on your feet, rubbing away all the dead bits of skin. Now stand up and exfoliate all over. Once you've done this, you will have to get out because the bath will feel like someone has dropped a bucket of sand in it. The ideal thing is to shower in order to rinse your hair and get rid of any exfoliating cream and face pack that is still lurking. If you can bring yourself to do so, finish off with a cold shower to get you tingling all over.

Once you're dry, rub in a mixture of moisturizer and toning cream/gel around your thighs, buttocks, and waist. You should not forget to moisturize your breasts on a regular basis either, as the skin around them is very sensitive and can get dry. Buy creams and lotions specifically designed for the breast and décolletage area—some are more effective than others, so make sure you buy them from a source that you can trust or get a recommendation from a friend. Dry your hair, maybe adding some leave-in conditioner for extra gloss.

Half an hour in the bathroom is far more relaxing than two hours slumped in front of the TV. If your libido has taken a nosedive recently, try actively relaxing with a nice bath rather than switching on the TV. You may well get a pleasant surprise. As you take positive steps to chill out, you'll find your interest in sex grows.

After a sexy bath, settle down to a sexy film. Check out IDEA 27, *Sex and the movies.*

Try another idea...

"Poetry is not the most important thing in life . . . I'd much rather lie in a hot bath reading Agatha Christie and sucking sweets."
DYLAN THOMAS

Defining idea...

105

How did it go?

Q   I don't have a tub. What can I do?

A   *Short of borrowing a friend's . . . you could still do a lot of the treatments and hop in and out of the shower. As far as steamy sex in the bathroom goes, the shower is, of course, far superior to the tub. Much more action, more options, and room to maneuver.*

Q   I don't have time for all this fiddling around. Is there a quicker way to baby perfect skin?

A   *Not really. Even if you're not a bath person, the point is that you fiddle around, investing time in yourself, making yourself feel cherished because it's utterly marvelous for making you feel and act sexier. If you don't want to take a bath, then spend the time nourishing your body and soul in other ways. This isn't time wasted. It's time spent nurturing yourself.*

25

Sporting chance

There is nothing quite as sexy as someone doing something well. And nowhere is this more pertinent than in the sporting arena.

Most of us play some sort of sport, or at least try to. It makes you feel good, keeps you in shape, and is a great way to meet other lithe, fit people. But what sets you apart from the crowd is if you're really excellent at something.

I once met a man who skied like a god. I remember we were in Switzerland somewhere and I had fallen over for the fiftieth time that morning. Weeping, I hauled my skis on to the cable car that was going down the mountain. Of course it was empty except for another two weeping heaps who couldn't face the humiliation and pain of getting down the mountain any other way. I stood at the back, looking at the view. Suddenly, my new boyfriend appeared, whizzing after the cable car,

Here's an idea for you...

A terrific shortcut to god-like sporting ability is to take up cycling. Once you've mastered a few basic skills, it is very easy to look like you know what you're doing on a bike. Added to that you have the bonus of a great buttock and thigh workout.

expertly leaping over moguls and grinning at me. At one point, he actually overtook us, and this was all back country. That was it. I was smitten.

A good sportsman or woman is very sexy. Someone who is confident and knows what they're doing is a turn-on. I mean who would ever have thought golf could become a sexy game? And then along came Tiger Woods and suddenly millions of bored housewives across the globe know what a hole-in-one is.

If you want to seduce the opposite sex with your sporting prowess, start practicing. General fitness is, of course, the first thing to work on. And if you're used to moving, e.g., running, swimming, cycling, rollerblading, or whatever, you will be more toned and fitter looking before you even start throwing a ball around. It's no good heaving your overweight frame on to the basketball court and expecting to look like Michael Jordan.

So your basic level of fitness is good. Now you just need to improve your golf swing, backhand, passing, breaststroke, whatever. The most obvious way is through coaching. This is especially effective in tennis and golf, where technique is important. For field sports, playing is really the only way to improve. You could go on a sports vacation to improve your skills. For example, Spain and Portugal are full of tennis schools where you spend a week doing not much more than hitting a ball. Or missing a ball, depending on how good you are.

Check out **IDEA 11, *Fitting in fitness*, for tips on how to stay fit always.**

Try another idea...

One tip for girls is not to go for the overly baggy, thick tracksuit look; it's never flattering. There are some loose fitting, thin cotton options around that are a much better idea. Short, tight tops look great, assuming you haven't got a huge midriff, with a little hooded sweatshirt or jacket to finish off the ensemble. Don't feel you need to show up looking like a color-coordinated page out of a catalog—that just makes everyone assume you've thought far too hard about it. Be casual but be classy.

"Pain is temporary, quitting lasts forever."
LANCE ARMSTRONG, cancer sufferer and record-breaking Tour de France winner

Defining idea...

How did it go?

Q   **I am just not the sporty type. No matter how hard I try I can't catch a ball. Is there any hope for me?**

A   *Develop an intellectual air and refuse to even go for a walk without a copy of* Ulysses *under your arm. Seriously, there are lots of sports you can try. Golf, riding, paragliding, windsurfing. You're not telling me you've tried everything are you?*

Q   **There must be more sedate ways of impressing the opposite sex; why waste the energy?**

A   *Of course there are. But as we all know, a good body is one of the single most important factors when it comes to being attractive. Sport is a great way of keeping in shape. Much more fun than the gym and potentially less expensive. We also know confidence is a big factor in sex appeal, and if you're good at something, even if it's darts, your confidence grows. So it's definitely worth the energy.*

26

Babes in toyland

Toys have a vital role to play in boosting confidence and making you feel sexier. And no, they're not for kids.

Women are realizing that sex toys guarantee them a much more satisfying love life and, funnily enough, when they're pretty sure they're going to have an orgasm, too, women are far more likely to want more sex.

Nowadays you don't have to go to some disreputable establishment to buy your "toys." There are sex shops all over the place—in some of the most respectable areas. There are also websites that make it very easy to shop without any risk of bumping into your neighbor.

Bed is one of the few places adults are still allowed to play, so you should take advantage. People have been using sex toys since the Stone Age. According to *The*

Here's an idea for you...

Go sex toy shopping with your lover. You can spend a happy hour browsing the shelves for toys that turn you on, as well as gels, books, strange underwear, and so forth. Go one morning and reserve the afternoon for sex.

Ann Summers Guide to Wild Sex and Loving, there are cave paintings depicting women using interesting-shaped pieces of flint to pleasure themselves. Luckily these days, any sex shop will provide you with something more comfortable made of rubber, plastic, or silicone. There is a huge amount of choice and only you can decide what best suits you and your sex life.

The most popular of all sex toys is the vibrator. These come in all sorts of shapes and (scary) sizes. A word on shape. It doesn't have to be phallic to make a woman come. Leather vibrators are the most realistic in terms of sensation in my opinion. Vibrators are not just to be used alone; they can also be used as an additional stimulus during sex. And not just for women; a friend of mine says her boyfriend loves his G-spot being stimulated with one. For those of you that don't know, a man's G-spot is a couple of inches into his anus. Your choice of dildo will depend on whether you want to go for a sexy look or just a functional one. There are very plain vibrators that you could pretend were useful for massaging a sore neck should your grandmother ever find them. Then there are the all-singing, all-dancing types with knobs that are so clearly used for nothing but sex games.

Pleasure balls are two balls connected by a cord, each containing ball bearings that move inside to create sexy sensations. As well as being good fun, they are perfect for toning the pelvic floor muscles and, as we all know, the stronger your pelvic floor muscles, the stronger your orgasms.

For more on sexy accessories and what to do with them see IDEA 47, *Tie me up, tie me down.*

Try another idea...

For men, the most popular toy is apparently the penis ring. It sounds rather painful to me but is designed to be slipped on before the penis is fully erect, thus trapping the blood in the erect penis and making the erection last for much longer than it otherwise would.

All these things are useful and fun accessories that can enrich your sex life. More importantly, they make you more confident and relaxed, which in turn makes you sexier. Someone who is not worried about a strap-on dildo is unlikely to be fazed by stripping seductively or massaging their lover.

"Deceive boys with toys, but men with oaths."
LYSANDER, ancient Greek general

Defining idea...

How did it go?

Q **I can't just get a huge dildo out in the middle of intercourse. She'll think I'm deranged, won't she?**

A *Perhaps, but you don't just have to pounce on her with it from nowhere. Tell her you have a sexy surprise for her and slowly introduce your new friend in your lovemaking. Make sure you know how to pleasure her with it before you start and don't be too heavy-handed.*

Q **Isn't this all a little perverted?**

A *Calm down. Nobody said you had to go for the double entry black mamba as a first toy. Try something a little innocuous, like some oil. You can even go for flavored massage oils. Then move on to something a bit riskier. Maybe a blindfold. From there you can progress to the vibrator and so forth. Try a sex game as well—they sell them in sex shops. They're a great way to get a little risqué with someone else, the game dictating what you do. This means you don't have to feel self-conscious when you're told to stimulate your partner's clitoris with a vibrator. You're only following orders!*

27

Sex and the movies

Films can inspire and turn you on. And I'm not talking porn films, the vast majority of which are a complete turn-off to most women and lots of men.

One moment that is consistently voted one of the sexiest scenes in film is Ursula Andress walking seductively out of the sea in the James Bond movie *Dr. No.*

It is an image that has endured, despite the fact that it was filmed more than forty years ago and films have gotten a lot more explicit since then. Bikini sales shot up when the film was released; every woman wanted to be Ursula and every man wanted to Andress her!

A recent survey of the top-ten sexy moments in film voted the above scene the winner. Also in the top ten are scenes from *Basic Instinct* and *Nine 1/2 Weeks*. There are valuable lessons in both on how to be sexy. Obviously, there are parts of *Basic Instinct* that you shouldn't try at home, but in one scene Sharon Stone made cinematic history by uncrossing her legs. Michael Douglas was powerless as the detective sent to investigate her. The famous "You know I'm not wearing any underwear" line had most of the males in the audience drooling. We can't all be as brash or as bold as

Here's an idea for you...

With your partner, compile a top-ten list of sexy moments on film. This is a great way to spend an evening in itself, going through all your old favorites and picking the ones you like best. Then set dates when you can plan and produce your own top-ten hot scenes.

Sharon Stone, but if you watch her carefully you can pick up some good tips.

Nine 1/2 Weeks is a sex lesson in itself. It may seem a bit dated twenty years down the line but is worth watching to pick up some great sexy tips. How many millions of couples all over the world raided their fridges after they'd seen it and started blindfolding each other? I couldn't look at a strawberry without blushing for weeks after it. How many women spent that year stripping to Joe Cocker's "You Can Leave Your Hat On"? Rarely, if ever, has a film inspired so much sex; it would be interesting to know if birth rates went up nine months from around the time it was released! Strangely enough, Mickey Rourke has never been sexy since. Kim Basinger goes from strength to strength (another great sexy film she's in is *L.A. Confidential*).

Films are essentially about escape and fantasies. They transport us to another world and they inspire us. Learn to use films to increase your own sexiness by watching and really observing how the leads behave.

Here are some films and scenes to pick up sexy tips from. Look at the way the actors and actresses behave, check out their clothes, their movements, their speech. Try to define what it is that makes them so sexy and see if you can copy it. And, of course, there's nothing to say you shouldn't re-create some of the steamiest scenes in the comfort of your own home.

- *The Fabulous Baker Boys*—Sparks fly over the piano between Michelle Pfeiffer and Jeff Bridges, very sexy. Check out the tension between the two of them throughout and the stunningly sexy piano scene where they almost make love through the song. It's a great lesson in mixing work and pleasure. Watch the film and if you have a piano, try to re-create the scene at home. Almost worth buying one for.

Check out how to be literary and sexy in IDEA 7, *Literal appeal.*

Try another idea...

- *Dangerous Liaisons*—More Michelle Pfeiffer. Bodice-ripping drama set in eighteenth-century France. A great lesson in the dangers of immoral love as well as how to look sexy in a corset! Some of the scenes are well worth trying to re-create, like the one where the wicked Valmont pens a letter to his victim using Uma Thurman's buttocks as a writing desk.

- *Sex, Lies, and Videotape*—The title says it all. Infidelity, lust, pervy filming, and sex. Very entertaining. And a good idea for some fun at home. Get out your video camera or just a normal stills camera if you don't have one. Make your own porn film. Just remember to put it away when you've finished so you don't mix it up with the one of your nephew's christening.

"I'm tired of all this nonsense about beauty being only skin deep. That's deep enough. What do you want—an adorable pancreas?"
JEAN KERR, playwright

Defining idea...

How did it go?

Q   **What about going for a romantic film instead?**

A   *Good idea. There's no reason why romantic can't be sexy, too. You may find that you feel uncomfortable watching overt sex scenes whereas something more subtle will get your imagination working and inspire sexy feelings.*

Q   **Why don't we just cut to the chase and go for porn?**

A   *Don't let me stop you. It is important that you choose something that turns you on. Some people like to see every bump and grind while others prefer something more subtle, so figure out where your tastes lie and (as long as it's legal) go for it.*

28

Location, location, location

There is no doubt that some cities, restaurants, shops, and bars are sexy and some are not. Just like people. So how do you know what's hot and what's not?

It's no good being a sex deity if you're surrounded by geeks. You need to get where the action is. You need to hang out with other sexy types. So where are they all?

Where you are can help to define how sexy you are—if you know where to hang out then you're already halfway to being sexy. If you feel a little lost on this subject then pick up some glossy travel magazines and women's magazines with travel sections. They normally pick the most luxurious spots and hot places to hang out. If you can't afford to go there at the moment then at least you can be well informed so you know where to save up for. Buy some classic travel books and read up on places you want to go or places you have dreamt about.

There are some obvious answers that you can come up with yourself. New York, for example, has to be one of the sexiest cities in the world. It is brash, vibrant, hip, and cool. As soon as you land you feel like you've walked on to a film set.

Here's an idea for you...

Have a look at the Hip Hotels Guide series for inspiration. The hotels are seriously beautiful and romantic.

There are countless hotel options. You can stay in the Carlyle, where JFK and Marilyn Monroe apparently had their trysts. Or the new Dream Hotel, the ultimate in New York cool. If money is not an issue then the hotel with the best location in New York is the Four Seasons, or try the Algonquin, which is also home to the $10,000 martini (a martini with a diamond at the bottom). The hip bars and restaurants in the city are dotted all over, but if you stick to Greenwich Village you can't go wrong.

Just the name Paris makes you think of sex (no, I don't mean Ms. Hilton and her video antics). It is possibly the most gorgeous place in the world and in the spring can turn the most levelheaded traveler into a sex goddess. A friend of mine was there on a business trip recently. "I don't know what came over me," she says. "But all of a sudden I was mentally undressing men in the street, in the bars and cafés. It was totally weird but great fun." There is nothing like a walk in the gardens of the Palais Royal to bring out the romantic beast in you.

But where to stay? The sexiest hotel is called the Hôtel Costes—supermodels hang out there along with pop royalty and other glitterati. Definitely the place to be seen, there is a spa and swimming pool totally lit with candles. The Hôtel Lancaster is apparently Ewan McGregor's favorite, and the Hôtel de Sers has the sexiest bathrooms and best view of the Eiffel Tower. None of these are cheap, but they're where the action is.

Shopping in Paris is sometimes even better than sex—there are lots of options but you should check out the various excellent department stores such as Galeries Lafayette and the Fauborg St. Honoré, home to the major designers.

Getting there is half the fun: check out IDEA 29, *The art of sexy travel.*

Try another idea...

Out of town, in southern France, the hot spot for all you sex gods is Nikki Beach, close to St. Tropez. This is where the jet set go to get a tan. Kate Moss loves it and Jude Law taught his children to swim there. You have to be thin and beautiful not to stand out from the crowd. But don't be intimidated. Think of it like a game of tennis, where you're playing someone that's better than you in order to improve your game. If you're surrounded by beautiful people then you will start looking good, too. You'll raise your game, you just can't help it. A bad hair day on Nikki Beach is just not an option.

Gwyneth Paltrow is very fond of the Esperanza Hotel on the Los Cabos beach in Mexico. It has a candlelit cliff-top restaurant and plunge pools on the balcony. Total heaven. Also in Mexico is the newly refurbished One&Only Palmilla, where John Travolta spent his fiftieth birthday with 300 of his closest friends. Bathrooms overlook the beach and suites come with butlers. If you get bored with the butler you can play golf on a twenty-seven-hole golf course designed by Jack Nicklaus.

"What is commonly called love, namely the desire of satisfying a voracious appetite with a certain quantity of delicate human flesh."
HENRY FIELDING

Defining idea...

How did it go?

Q These are all luxury spots for film stars and rich people. What about us normal people?

A *Well, what would be the fun in a chapter on neighborhood bars? Even if you can't afford to stay in these places, you can still enjoy them. Go for a drink, a swim, or just a snoop.*

Q I'm single at the moment. Is it worth going alone?

A *Of course. Traveling alone is a great way to meet people. And you should in no way feel bad about being alone. When you go out to eat, make sure you get a table right in the middle of the action, order a bottle of wine, and watch the world go by. I once watched a single man in a restaurant join a very attractive single lady when she was eating her dessert and they left together after dinner. Talk about speed dating.*

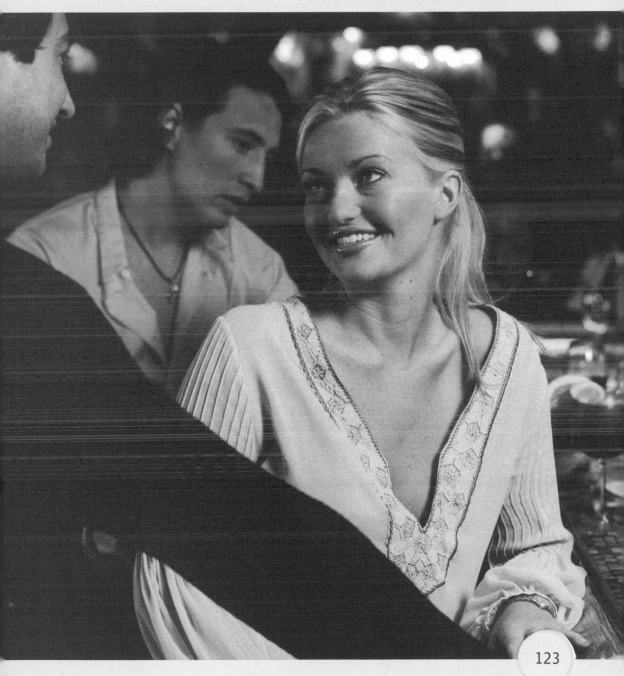

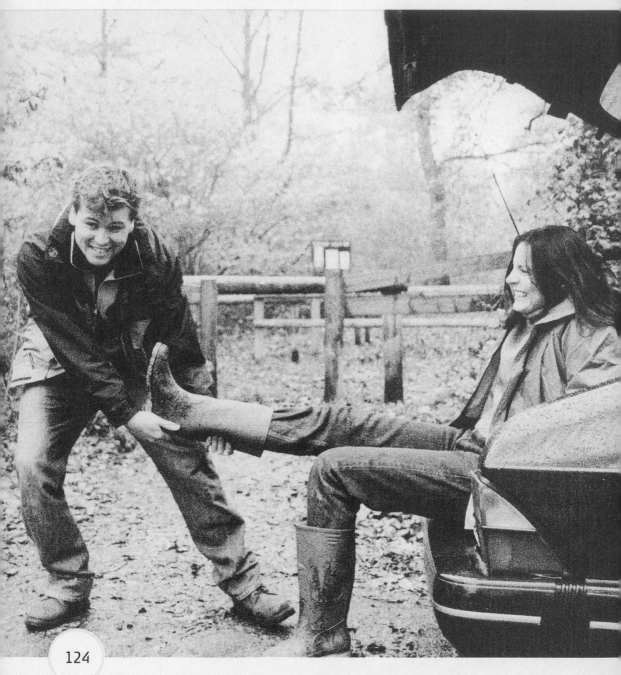

29

The art of sexy travel

Getting there is half the fun. Especially if you know how to travel well. You'd be surprised at what a difference getting there in style makes in how you feel once you arrive.

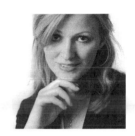

There are some essential tips you need to follow if you don't want to arrive looking like something the cat dragged in and feeling even worse.

Flying wreaks havoc with your whole body. You get dehydrated, tired, and arrive looking pasty and ill. There are several ways to lessen the pain. If you can possibly afford it, fly first class especially for long journeys. If you fly first class you will at least have been able to distance yourself from drunken fellow travelers and get some sleep. And you'll get to relax in the VIP lounge beforehand. The whole first-class experience just makes getting there so much more enjoyable.

If (like most of us) you're thinking "dream on" then there are other options. You can try to talk your way to an upgrade—but be clever and be original. Most airline staff will have heard the "it's our honeymoon" line hundreds of times. Or you can call around to travel agents or trawl online for bargain seats. You can also try courier

Here's an idea for you...

Any little testers you get you should save for when you are traveling. That way you will always have a good moisturizer or face pack on hand. Any time you see good quality shampoo in travel sizes, snap it up. Washing your hair in most hotels' shampoo is just not an option. It leaves your hair feeling like it's been washed in nail polish remover.

companies; they will often pay a big chunk of your ticket in return for delivery of a package, meaning that you may be able to afford the upgrade. It does pay to arrive early, too, as there is more chance that you will be able to get emergency exit seats, which at least have extra legroom.

There are things you can do to arrive looking sexier whatever class you're in. If you are on a long-haul flight and the lights are out, put on a moisturizing face pack for the night. In the morning, wash it off and put on a moisturizing lotion to brighten your face up. Take lots of hand cream and some of your favorite scent to spray on when you land. (Just make sure the bottles are small enough to take on board with you.) Don't forget your hairbrush and breath freshener, too. If you're on the flight overnight then changing your underwear just before you land, as well as your top, will make you feel fresher. And remember not to succumb to the temptations of that glass of wine or gin and tonic (no matter how bored you get). Flying dehydrates you and alcohol makes it worse. Sip water all the way through the journey. Try to eat healthily. That usually means avoiding airline food. Pack your own picnic.

Trains are a great way to travel. In fact, they are a great place to have sex as well. First class doesn't cost that much extra and it's really worth it. You arrive feeling pampered and refreshed instead of harassed. There is something so much more civilized about first-class travel. Look out for special first-class offers. For example, in France they sometimes sell $200 tickets between Paris and the south first-class. A bargain; you arrive at Nikki Beach ready for action.

Try going by car, sexily. Check out IDEA 33, *Va-va-vroom-vroom.*

Try another idea...

Driving can be a good way to get there if you can take time to meander through the countryside, stopping off at charming little hotels along the way. Convertibles are very sexy. To avoid arriving looking like you've been dragged there wear a head scarf and some sunglasses. Very Jackie O. However, you may well look and feel better if you hire a car with air-conditioning. Convertibles work best for short trips, not days of travel. And remember, linen is not a good option when traveling: you will arrive looking like you need a good iron.

"For my part, I travel not to go anywhere, but to go. I travel for travel's sake. The great affair is to move."
ROBERT LOUIS STEVENSON

Defining idea...

How did it go?

Q **What about dealing with all the stress of travel? How do I arrive looking and feeling sexy if I've had to deal with all of that?**

A *Leave yourself loads of time, especially if you are traveling with children. Planning far ahead and, most importantly, leaving tons of extra time to get to the airport is the surest way of ensuring that everything goes smoothly.*

Q **What do I do if I'm on my way to meet my lover and I fall in love with someone else on the plane?**

A *Ah yes, a common dilemma. You could try joining the mile-high club then and there and getting it out of your system. Failing that, swap numbers and get in touch at a later date. Dumping someone at the airport is not a nice thing to do. If you must, at least wait until you get to a place where they can make an escape. A rather evil male friend of mine once dumped someone on the Paris metro by handing her his metro ticket with: "It's been real, it's over," written on it. What a charmer. But at least she could get off at the next stop.*

30

Sex on the brain

A good sex life is the key to being incredibly sexy, and fantasies have a large role to play in ensuring that.

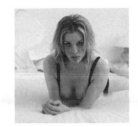

*Feeding the mind stimulates the body.
Be bold.*

For a lot of people, especially women, sex is as much in the mind as in the more obvious erogenous zones. To be sexy their minds need to be in tune with their bodies. And fantasy helps that enormously.

A friend of mine told me all about an Italian boyfriend she once had who was great at fantasies. During foreplay he would whisper fantasy situations in her ear. "Imagine we are at the opera," he would say. "We are alone in the royal box. I am sitting behind you and I start caressing you, putting my hands under your dress, feeling the tops of your stockings. Everyone is watching the stage, we are trying to be as quiet as possible. I ease you off your chair and onto my lap . . ." You can imagine the rest. She found this irresistible and discovered it was his storytelling she missed most when they split up. She never met anyone else who did the same thing and really didn't feel she could ask them to.

In terms of sexual fantasies, men and women are very different. According to one survey I read, men's most common fantasy involves a close friend. This just shows

Here's an idea for you... **Research has shown that short bursts of sexy thoughts throughout the day have a cumulative effect on your sex drive. Whenever you have a spare moment think about the last time you had sex or what you plan to do with your partner that night. Priming your mind primes your body. It makes you want sex more—and that's very sexy.**

what faithless beasts they are, always eyeing up your girlfriends! Women on the other hand, mostly fantasize about their partners. And they don't even fantasize about them doing something perverted, they fantasize about them behaving totally normally in bed. Come on girls, you can do better than that! You shouldn't feel guilty about fantasizing about people other than your partner. Bringing someone new into your sex life, in mind if not in body, can help boost your libido without causing any waves in the relationship.

Here are some interesting ideas—see if any of them grab you.

One survey found that the beach worked for women. Lying naked on a hot, deserted beach gets us going. Sex with an entire sports team excited some, and women also like the idea of a stranger in the night who is going to take them to some seedy hotel room and pleasure them for hours. The most popular one though was the thought of being tied up and dominated.

For men the most popular fantasy is the age-old "sex with two women at the same time." The most common scenario was having oral and genital sex at the same time. Another popular one is watching two women having sex. In fact, anything to do with two women seems to work for most men.

There is no getting away from the fact that men love lesbian fantasies. A friend of mine regularly narrates her boyfriend a fantasy situation involving her and her best friend. Her

If you want to make fantasy reality, why not spice up your life with IDEA 39?

Try another idea...

boyfriend loves it. The more graphic the detail, the better. And my friend loves it, too. "I think it's by far the best way to try a bit of lesbianism," she says. One survey I read concluded that 75 percent of women had a desire to try out lesbianism at least once. Don't forget that the lesbian thing could make you that much sexier in the eyes of your loved one. Sexiness is not just about looking good but about having the imagination and the confidence to break some boundaries.

For those of you who need to kick-start your imagination, use fantasies to give you a basic idea and build on that. Why not construct the narrative with your partner and see where it leads. Don't forget to set boundaries beforehand so that you each know what the other is happy with (if thinking of someone you know is a total turn-off for one of you, figure that out at the outset).

"Fantasy is often better than reality."
ANONYMOUS

Defining idea...

Q   Fantasies sound dangerous to me—won't this all end in tears?

A   *Fantasies are daydreams, or wishful thinking. They are really, completely, totally harmless and actually healthy. In the way your dreams sometimes sort out your problems, fantasies can help you iron out thoughts and issues you're trying to deal with. They also enable us to act out things we can't act out in real life. As adults we suppress our imagination during the day. Let it go, but maybe not when you're driving.*

Q   I'm far too embarrassed to talk about my fantasies. Any tips?

A   *Just go for it—he'll love it. It's not like he doesn't have them. Why don't you sit down and compile a list of fantasies you'd like to play out with each other? Assuming it's your partner you're fantasizing about, that is.*

31

Get the massage?

Just the word *massage* can make you go all warm. It is a fantastic way to create intimacy and surprisingly easy to do.

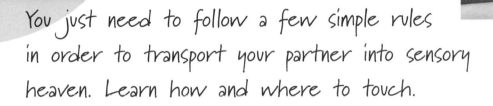

You just need to follow a few simple rules in order to transport your partner into sensory heaven. Learn how and where to touch.

Start at the top. Using your middle and index fingers gently massage the temples with circular motions. Don't neglect the scalp. Use all your fingers to massage it, again in circular motions, varying the pressure depending on how your partner likes it. The face should be paid special attention, especially the area around the mouth where the nerve endings are very near the surface. Gently smooth your thumb over the eyebrows and closed eyelids. You could supplement this part of the massage with some gentle butterfly kisses or fluttering your eyelashes on your partner's face.

Once you move on to the neck and shoulders you need to sit astride your loved one's buttocks. Whether you do this in the nude or not is up to you, but naked certainly increases the intimate aspect of the massage. Be careful not to put too much weight on your partner. Guys, in particular, may want to take some of the weight on their knees. Gently knead the flesh at the base of the neck, putting pressure on it with your thumbs, which, again, should move in circular motions.

Here's an idea for you...

Try Thai massage—a slightly crazy but fun idea. You need to do this in a bathroom, as it involves a lot of soap and water. Basically, the woman lathers herself up with soap and when she's really soapy and slippery she lies on top of her partner and writhes around, thereby giving him a full body massage. The process can be reversed but the man would have to take his weight off the woman.

You must be sensitive here to the amount of pressure your partner enjoys. This is the area where all the stress collects and so can be extremely sensitive. If your partner likes a deep massage try small karate chops with both hands along the top of the shoulders, which is very good for releasing tension.

The back is a wonderful arena. You can move with large sweeping movements from the buttocks upward, then work your way down the spine, pressing along each vertebra with your thumbs. With plenty of oil on your hands, start from the spine and almost flick your hands away from it, releasing tension as you work your way down.

Now we reach the buttocks and here's where you can really get going. Use a bit of pressure, the extra flesh here can take it. To get really deep, knead the flesh with your palms. Don't neglect the sacrum. This little area just above the bottom crease is extremely sensitive.

For the legs, you need to start just above the ankle and using the palm of your hand to push all the way up to the buttocks. The inner thigh is an incredibly erogenous zone so you should gently massage that as well. Don't forget the feet. Start by holding the top of one foot with one hand and gently rotating it with the other.

The reflexology point directly linked to sex drive is on the inside of the foot about half a centimeter below the anklebone—so make sure you pay special attention to that.

A massage after a bath is divine. Discover IDEA 24, *The art of the sexy bath*.

Try another idea...

Now you need to roll your partner over and focus on the stomach and chest. Guys should work around the breasts in gentle circular movements, but don't forget to finish off with a gentle nipple caress, either with your mouth or your fingers. Try gentle sweeping movements on the stomach, too, focusing on the lower stomach (very sensitive). Tease them slightly by moving down as far as you dare. In certain kinds of massage parlors they often ask if you would like a "special massage." You can offer the same if the mood takes you.

Remember to have plenty of massage oils on hand to make the experience more sensual. Choose your oil to go with your mood. Lavender is relaxing, rose is romantic, sandalwood is used to treat a low libido. Mix a small amount of the essential oil with a base oil, such as sweet almond oil—most essential oils should not be applied to the skin in their undiluted form.

"'Where should one use perfume?' a young woman asked. 'Wherever one wants to be kissed,' I said."
COCO CHANEL

Defining idea...

How did it go?

Q **I could read about this in any old massage book. How about some sexier tips?**

A   *You asked for it. Try a genital massage. Sound weird? If you're a guy then start by dribbling a little warmed (not hot!) oil over her genitals, letting it trickle slowly down. Trace the contours of her labia and the sensitive skin on her inner thigh. If you're female then you should start with the same oil treatment, warming it in your hands first, and start massaging around the penis. Explore the whole area, the balls and the scrotum. Don't focus on the penis to start with. Eventually you can start caressing his penis, using both hands. Remember, this is not a place to apply pressure.*

Q **Are there any accessories I should use when I massage?**

A   *The most important thing is oil, and there are any number of oils available. You can also buy heat-activated massage oil that warms up when you use it. During a massage you can also experiment with some sex toys—a vibrator, for example. Start using it as a massage tool and move on from there to more erotic uses.*

32

The tan commandments

Having a tan makes you look thinner, healthier, and sexier. There really is no downside—lookswise. But healthwise, you have to prepare yourself for the beach.

So we've all heard about the dental floss look on Copacabana Beach. That minuscule, almost invisible bikini all those hot Brazilian chicks wear.

But how would you look in one of those while sunning yourself at the shore? (An unlikely thought, in itself.) It's no good just exposing that flabby white flesh and hoping you'll leave the beach looking like Halle Berry. You'll look more like a boiled lobster. You need to prepare yourself for the suntan and this can take weeks of advance planning.

You need to prepare your skin, especially if it's fair. Some people take beta carotene pills for a few weeks before they go on vacation. This substance can help you go brown and can be found in carrots and other brightly colored vegetables as well as the pills. You should exfoliate before you expose your skin to the sun. This removes dead skin and makes the tan more even. Try body brushing or use exfoliating creams. Once on vacation be sure to put on sunscreen before tanning and not just

Here's an idea for you...

Try bleaching the body hair that you're holding on to before you start sunbathing. That way they will be lovely and blonde, making you look even more tanned and gorgeous, and you won't be self-conscious about them. Jolen Cream Bleach is the best one.

when you've burnt (when it's too late). Sunscreens should be applied about half an hour before you go outside. During the first few days, limit your tanning sessions to twenty minutes and avoid the sun between 11:30 and 2:30. You must moisturize all the time, use a good after-sun product in the evening, and keep piling on that cream during the day. The sun drinks the moisture from your skin. It also removes collagen, the substance that gives your skin elasticity. So you need to make sure you take plenty of vitamin C while on vacation, as your body can't produce collagen without it.

Tanned skin is damaged skin and the more you expose the skin to the sun the more damaged it will become over time. No wonder so many people swear by a fake tan. Products are improving all the time so if you purchase and apply wisely you should be able to avoid the dreaded streaks. To ensure even color remember to exfoliate before applying the fake tan and apply sparingly to areas like knees and elbows. Either wear special fake tanning gloves or wash the palms of your hands thoroughly after applying.

You also need to prepare your body. This means a diet and a strict exercise regime at least two months before you plan to wear that dental floss. In terms of what to wear on the beach, this obviously depends on who you're vacationing with and where you're going. In Rio, one can definitely get away with a minuscule bikini. They wear practically nothing there, even the women without great bodies. Somehow they get away with it, they move well, are tanned and confident.

So where do you show off your new tan? Find out in IDEA 28, *Location, location, location.*

Try another idea...

The only thing to avoid is looking cheap. You can always wear the minuscule bikini while lying around trying to catch the rays, but cover up with a sarong when you're wandering around. A classic swimsuit can be extremely elegant and sexy, too—don't assume that in the beachwear stakes, less is always more.

Don't forget your hair. Seawater and sun can take their toll. Give it a deep conditioning treatment every time you wash it. Comb the conditioner through carefully and wrap your hair in a hot towel. If you're trying to go blonde, squeeze lemon juice into it for some natural and cheap highlights. But don't forget to condition it well every day, as lemon juice has a drying effect.

"Summertime and the livin' is easy."
HEYWARD and GERSHWIN, songwriters

Defining idea...

How did
it go?

Q   **Can't I just cover myself in oil for that really sexy look?**

A   *Of course—once the sun has gone down. But during the day you need a proper sunscreen. Oil will attract the sun and you'll literally fry. If you live in a warm climate (or even during the summer months) you should wear a moisturizer with an SPF of at least 15 to protect your face. It is recommended that you throw away old sunscreens and buy new ones every year since the effect of the heat will make them basically useless the following season. A bit expensive, but there are so many new, improved products out that you might want a change anyway.*

Q   **If I wear suntan lotion every time, I'm never going to get brown in two weeks. How can I look gorgeous?**

A   *But you might look better at fifty. Sun-damaged skin looks rough, red, and puffy. And that's before we start on the risk of skin cancer. No one wants to be a killjoy but there's evidence that binge tanning—really going for it for just a few weeks a year—carries more risk of cancer than exposure over a longer period.*

33

Va-va-vroom-vroom

Sports cars and sex appeal have gone hand in velvet glove since the first car salesman realized he could put the words "throbbing," "racy," and "curvy" into a single sentence.

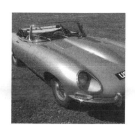

Cars can be very sexy, there's no denying it, and if you don't happen to have Lamborghini looks yourself, you can always borrow a little racy appeal from your four-wheeled friend.

A friend of mine has always had a convertible Porsche. He is not great looking, but says that women actually get into the car when he stops at traffic lights. "It's extraordinary," he told me. "They have no shame." A man in a Porsche has become a bit of a cliché (you mean you've never heard of the male menoporsche?), but there is no denying that cars can help a man's sex appeal.

The trick to car-isma is not about being able to afford that dream machine (although that obviously works for some), it's about looking like you were born behind the wheel of one, even if your finances are more Ford Fiesta than Ferrari Testarossa.

Everyone (and especially every man) has their own dream machine hit parade. Just a few of my own favorites would include:

Here's an idea for you... **If you can't afford any of these cars then join a car share. The best ones own a pool of vehicles and your annual fee buys you time-shares. You're a part-owner, so you'll come across as a connoisseur, not a con man. Try the Internet or your national classic car magazines for club details.**

- E-Type Jaguar—so sublimely sexy that even Austin Powers gets the girl in one. Possibly the most phallic car ever made. What's not to like?

- Lamborghini P400 Miura—if your date shows up in one of these you know he's not only fabulously rich, but a connoisseur. Only a handful of these exist; most of them have been written off by playboys on the twisting roads above Monaco.

- Bentley Arnage Red Label—a massive British vehicle, a cross between a dreadnought battleship and a steelworks. Can reach massive speeds, but not a good place to keep your blow-dry in place.

- Aston Martin DB9—the latest evocation of this legend from the manufacturers of James Bond's famous machine-gun equipped DB5. The DB9 has the lines of a film star and the power of a small aircraft. Caution: Any man driving one is likely to think more about the car than you.

- Ferrari Dino—if Sophia Loren was a car, this is the one she would be.

- Mini Cooper—an extraordinary piece of design, popular with everyone from John Lennon to Michael Caine's bank mob in *The Italian Job*. It's enjoying a revival now—waiting lists are six months for the convertible model.

- Alfa Romeo Spider—think Dustin Hoffman in *The Graduate*.

Think a little about what these cars are saying and see if you can say it in other ways. Obviously, if what you want to say is that you are hugely rich and you aren't, you may have a problem. If what you want to say is that you identify with these cars' sense of elegance or ruggedness, then you've got something you can work with whatever your budget. A convertible is just a car without a roof, but any woman in any convertible who sports '50s sunglasses and a head scarf instantly becomes Grace Kelly in *To Catch a Thief*. Just beware of long scarves and cars with spoked wheels, in case you instantly become Isadora Duncan instead.

Guys, remember that stubble is pretty much required when stepping out of a four-wheel off-roader. On the other hand there's a lot of eye-catch factor to be found by playing the unexpected. Think Brosnan's Bond straightening his tie from the driver's seat of a tank. Don't forget that almost any car is made sexier by the addition of a half-bottle of champagne and two flutes in the glove compartment.

Ultimately, of course, the whole point of a sexy car is to have sex in it. Get in touch with your inner teenager and go for it. What fun: The leather seats, the windows steaming up, the unexpected encounter with the hand brake, indeed the sheer challenge, makes sex in a car unforgettable.

If you would prefer to let somebody else do the driving while you look fabulous and enjoy the scenery take a look at IDEA 29, *The art of sexy travel.*

Try another idea...

"Why are women wearing perfumes that smell like flowers? Men don't like flowers. I've been wearing a great new scent guaranteed to attract men. It's called New Car Interior."
RITA RUDNER, comedian

Defining idea...

How did it go?

Q   **If I live on beans and water for six months I'll just about be able to afford four wheels and an engine—how do you do sexy on a budget?**

A   *Whoever you are your image will be greatly enhanced if you travel in something cool. It doesn't have to be hugely expensive. On my own sexy list there are also cute little cars like the Mini Cooper and the Deux Chevaux. The thing is not to go for something horribly ugly. This includes almost any car that is white (not a good look) or anything that smacks of flashiness, like go-faster stripes and oversized tires. But any car with character has sex appeal.*

Q   **I hanker after the wind in my hair, the sun on my visor, the flies on my teeth . . . any tips here?**

A   *Ah yes, motorcycles. Some girls like them. In fact, some girls adore them. But wind in the hair means good-bye hairstyle. The alternative "helmet head" look is only suitable for those of us with '60s bob cuts (or shaved heads—it takes all types). Most importantly of all, however cool they may look, motorcycles will only ever appeal to a minority of the population. So you are limiting the pool of people who are going to find your wheels incredibly sexy.*

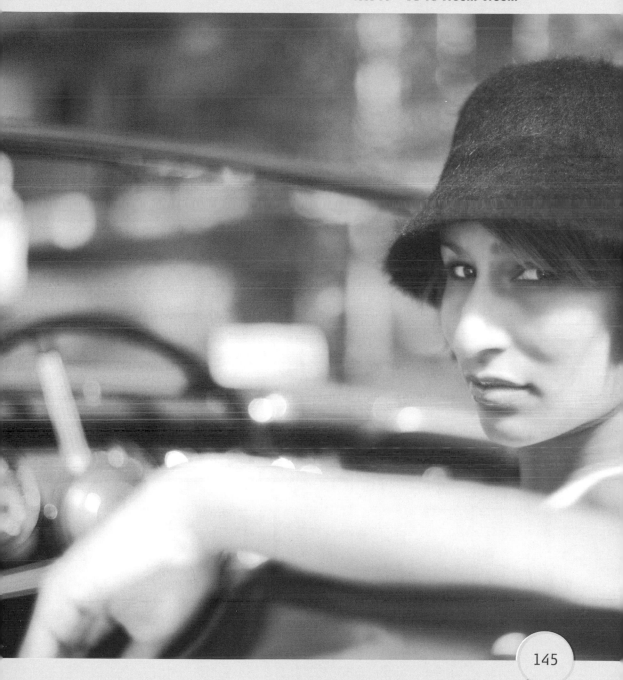

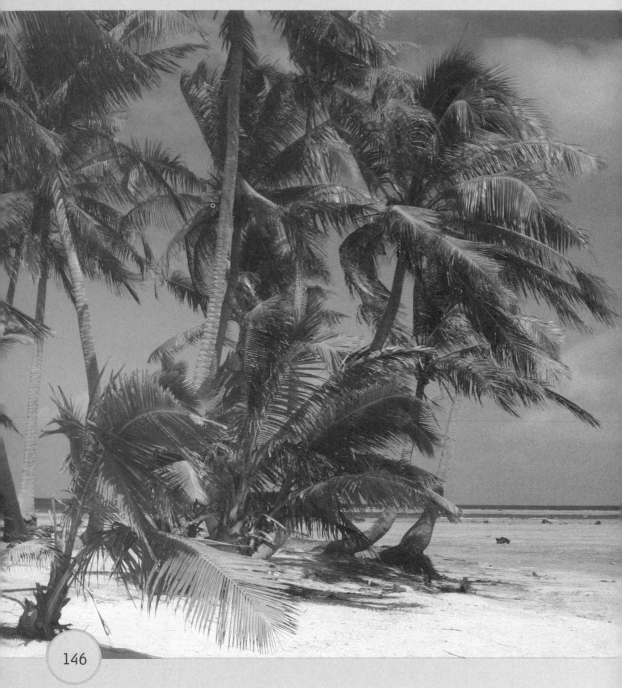

34

Wow, voyager!

Let's face it. If you tell someone you're going to Rio, they think sex. If you tell them you're going to Brussels, they don't. Like people, countries have their own identity and some of them are sexy, some are not.

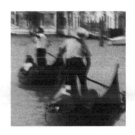

So how do you choose where to go for the ultimate sexy trip?

It is very important when choosing your sexy trip that you go for somewhere that conjures up sexy images for both of you. You need the right surroundings to bring out the sexy beast in you and your partner.

Short of ideas? I think one of the reasons that Rio is so sexy is the climate. It is literally steamy; hot, humid, and sunny. Rio oozes sex. It seems to be on everyone's mind. Even the way they walk and talk there is sexy. The people are very open and kind. The best time to go for a truly steamy time is in their summer, between November and March. The only place to stay is the best hotel in town: the incomparable Copacabana Palace Hotel on Copacabana Beach. It is expensive, but it is to die for and there is nothing like a luxury hotel to bring out the best in you. If you're being looked after and pampered then you can focus on being sexy. At the Copacabana they have a massage service that actually comes to your room.

Here's an idea for you... **If you're off on your honeymoon, instead of wedding presents get your friends to put money into a honeymoon fund. You should talk to your travel agent and see what honeymoon offers they have. The wedding magazines are also full of good ideas and bargains.**

A woman shows up with a foldable bed, oil, and towels, so after the massage you can just roll onto your bed, fully oiled up and relaxed.

It helps to be warm. I am half Swedish and although it's a lovely place, I wouldn't recommend Stockholm in November as a sex-on-the-beach destination. Warmth is so much easier to deal with and you can wear far fewer clothes. Strolling down a beach in a bikini and a sarong is a lot more conducive to feeling sexy than shivering in a hailstorm. Although, if you get it right, a skiing holiday can also be very sexy. The cold air and open fireplaces can be an extremely potent combination.

You don't have to go for a full-blown vacation to get benefits. The dirty weekend is a great invention. Imagine just going away to be dirty. The fact that you've made the decision to do just that will make you feel sexy in itself. You are there to enjoy each other and nothing is going to get in your way; no children, no phones, no washing up. What could be better? You can just focus on the three most important things in anyone's dirty weekend itinerary: drinking, eating, and having sex.

For the ideal dirty weekend, book into a luxury hotel with a pervy twist, like the Gran Hotel La Florida in Barcelona, just to take time out to be together. This hotel not only has magnificent views over the city but a room with a mirror in the ceiling. Bathrooms are essential when booking a hotel room for a sexy break. They should be big and have a romantic freestanding Victorian bath. Just the sight of one of those is enough to inspire sexy thoughts. Four-poster beds are also fun. Before you book the hotel go through a checklist of what you're after and make sure they have it all.

When you're away from your usual routine with someone else taking care of all the boring chores, it's easier to feel more in the mood, of course. Stress is the enemy of sexy; the more stressed we are, the lower our libido is likely to be. A place can be sexy simply because it's different, because you're away from the worries and stresses of home and work. You suddenly feel liberated and free, able to be yourself and let yourself go. But if foreign trips are just not possible right now, remember that the reason they're so good for your sex life is the reduced stress. So do that, or settle for a weekend somewhere in the United States. It might be enough to give you that feeling of escape.

If you don't feel like traveling, go for the sexy evening in. More on that in IDEA 23, There's no place like home.

Try another idea...

"The great advantage of a hotel is that it's a refuge from home life."
GEORGE BERNARD SHAW

Defining idea...

How did it go?

Q I can't afford one of those luxury hotels you talked about, let alone the flight to Rio.

A *Look on the Internet for bargain packages: you might find there are some great deals with flight, food, and accommodation included. Even the best hotels sometimes have cheap deals. Talk to your local travel agent and tell them what you're after, they might be able to help.*

Q What do I do if the weather is a washout? That makes it hard to feel sexy.

A *Use your imagination. Sex in the rain is not a bad option if it's not too cold. If you're somewhere tropical, swimming in the rain is actually quite enjoyable and you'll have the beach to yourself.*

35

Glamour—how to get it

As my father once said, "There is nothing original since God said 'Let there be light.' " So don't feel bad about stealing tips from others and using them to increase your sex appeal.

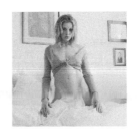

Most people agree on what is sexy, with slight variations. Look to those who epitomize these qualities. Adapt them for yourself and you can't fail to be sexier.

Sean Connery may not be the most beautiful man around but he is consistently voted one of the sexiest, even at his advanced age. I think this has to do with his manner. He is a real man's man, but one who knows how to treat a woman like a lady, something which is still incredibly attractive to women and should not be underestimated. I have yet to meet a woman who would be offended if a man opened a door for her, carried her suitcase, or paid for dinner. So don't let all that political correctness put you off: Be a gentleman. A friend of mine told me she fell in love with her husband the first time she met him because he was the only male in the room to stand up when she walked in. In fact, she went to bed with him that same night, and fifteen years later they are still together.

Here's an idea for you...

If you're a man, do your crunches every day, at least 250. Just roll out of bed and onto the floor first thing every morning. Don't forget to work the lower and upper abs for that seriously hot look. You work the lower abs by doing crunches that involve both the upper and lower body; basically your elbows and knees meet over your stomach. For the upper body just straight sit-ups will do.

Female role models abound. If you watch Marilyn's films, she is almost invariably vulnerable and sweet. This brings out the macho instinct in men who love to look after a doe-eyed nymph. But remember Marilyn's on-screen dippy image was far from the bright and intelligent woman she really was. At the other end of the spectrum from Marilyn we have sassy women like Sharon Stone and Halle Berry. Tips from these two would include looking great at all times (I dread to think the amount of tricep dips Halle Berry must do) and being perfectly done up as well as oozing confidence and know-how. Catherine Zeta Jones is an interesting combination of the two types and in my view has got the sex appeal thing totally dead-on. She has proper curves, classic feminine long black hair, but is totally in control of things. I suppose it may also have something to do with the roles she plays, but even just purely in the looks department she has combined sexy and sassy extremely effectively. Julia Roberts is a very sexy Hollywood star who is always smiling. The one thing you can learn from her is to look happy.

For you guys, it all depends on the image you want, but contemporary stars that are generally seen as sexy include Brad Pitt and George Clooney. The one thing they have is an attractive cheekiness that is irresistible. Brad has the famous washboard stomach (more on that on the opposite page), and George looks as if he's lived life to the fullest and not forgotten anything he's learned along the way. And that's nearly irresistible.

If you can't copy anyone, be yourself, but with added spark. Find out how to develop your sexy sense of humor in IDEA 44, *Make 'em laugh.*

Try another idea...

"*I have never yet seen anyone whose desire to build up his moral power was as strong as sexual desire.*"
CONFUCIUS

Defining idea...

153

Q   **I look nothing like any of these people.**

A   *They don't look like themselves before the makeup artists, lighting, and computer people have finished retouching their images. But what they do have is charisma and confidence. That comes with practice. You can copy it.*

Q   **What about tips from ordinary people?**

A   *Absolutely. If you find someone attractive, try to define why and then copy that particular attribute. There are lots of things we see every day that are sexy; the key is to be on the lookout and aware of them. Then you can copy them.*

36

Aging sexily

**These days forty is like twenty—only with better clothes.
Your sex appeal can be just as potent at forty as at twenty.**

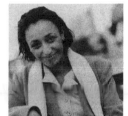

Mrs. Robinson's seduction of Benjamin in
the film *The Graduate* epitomized the
fascination of the older woman. She is
sophisticated, confident, alluring, all-knowing—
all things that make her extremely sexy and
attractive.

Remember that opposites attract. Young men like older women. There is nothing as
boring as a young man when you're young and an old man when you're old. A
forty-two-year-old friend of mine recently came back from a trip to St. Tropez where
she spent a week having wild sex with a twenty-year-old on his year off between
school and college. It might be a cliché, but sex with an attractive older woman is
most young men's idea of a good time.

Here's an idea for you... **Use your fortieth birthday as an excuse for a makeover. Take a day off to go to a spa, relax, get a facial and a manicure. Get a new haircut and then go to your favorite shop and buy yourself four new outfits; one for every decade. Re-create yourself every "0" birthday from now on.**

Similarly, you men should take comfort in the story of a sixty-year-old male friend of mine. He is going out with someone in her twenties and she is crazy for him. "I find men my own age so dull," she told me. "With James I feel like I'm learning something." So there you have it. Young men want to learn about sex, young women want to learn about life.

Of course you can also sleep with people your own age. Middle-aged sex needn't be dull. Just look at the film stars that have hit forty—Brad Pitt among them. Not many women would say no to a night with him. Catherine Deneuve is glorious at sixty. A friend of mine in her early fifties was recently on a business trip in Budapest with her boss, also in his mid-fifties. They got drunk and acted like teenagers, having sex all night. "I felt great," she told me. "It made me realize that essentially we don't change that much. We might get older on the outside but we're the same on the inside." Go on, get in touch with your inner teenager.

Older skin and the older body need to be looked after more carefully. The good news is that by the time you're forty you're in a better position to afford all those creams and lotions you need to retain a youthful glow. Remember that you will have to be more regimented about skin care—regular facials, cleansing morning and evening, exfoliation, cellulite treatment, and so forth. You will also need to be more careful in the sun.

As we have seen throughout this book, sexiness has a lot to do with confidence. And at forty-plus you are a lot more confident than you were at twenty. You are more secure in your own skin and you are probably more aware of what you want in bed than you were twenty years ago.

If you're feeling a bit old and blue, pamper yourself. Try IDEA 48, *Preparation, preparation, preparation*.

Try another idea...

Scientists have finally started to dismiss the midlife crisis. New research suggests that the forties are fun and a time of happiness. They have identified an emotional growth spurt that makes people more relaxed and easier to spend time with; in other words once you're forty, you're better company. "We start relaxing and enjoying life and other people fully only when we hit our late thirties," says Samuel Gosling, a British psychologist.

And the fun doesn't stop at forty. Research shows that people grow more content as they grow older. Chances are you'll be a lot happier at sixty-five than you were at twenty-five. Being happy helps you radiate allure.

"Whatever wrinkles I got, I enjoyed getting them."
AVA GARDNER

Defining idea...

How did it go?

Q   This is great, but my body is sagging. What can I do about it?

A   *Join the club. And as I know, the only answer is to work at it. This is where daily lunges, push-ups, and sit-ups are an essential part of your routine. For women, make yourself and self-maintenance a priority. Also, you need to stop abusing your body as you did in your twenties. Heavy drinking and smoking are out.*

Q   So am I safe to pounce on a young person I have the hots for?

A   *It depends on how closely connected you are to them. If you'll never meet again, do what you like. But be wary of the true Mrs. Robinson scenario. A friend of mine was once horribly attracted to the son of a family friend. She told me she thought he felt the same way about her. But when it came to acting on this impulse she was worried that if she lunged he would keel back in horror and tell her he was going to call his parents, followed by the police! An unlikely scenario, as my friend is a gorgeous blond Swede. However, you need to be careful. Learn to pick up on body language and other signs and don't take light flirting as a sign that they want to sleep with you. And even if all that is in place, it might still be best to avoid children of friends. It's a bit close to home.*

37

Absence makes the heart grow fonder

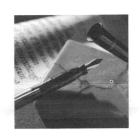

After our first date, my husband sent me a postcard. I can't remember what the picture was but his handwriting was so beautiful that I fell in love on the spot.

In the past, whole relationships were conducted via letters. Expressing yourself in the written word is one way to keep in touch with a loved one when you're away and can be extremely sexy.

Now that we live in the age of emails and cell phones, the simple old letter doesn't really figure in much. But it's amazing how romantic it is. Next time you're away from your loved one, try writing him a letter telling him how much you miss him and describing what you would like to be doing if you were with him.

Here's an idea for you...

If your handwriting is appallingly bad (like mine) then try to improve it. Slow your writing down. Develop a test sentence that you write every day at the top of a page. Compare and contrast to see what progress you have made.

Emails are a great way to keep in touch. You can flirt in emails as the exchange is almost immediate, like a conversation. Cyber romances have taken over where pen pals left off. A friend of mine had an incredibly intense relationship with a man she met on the Internet. "We became obsessed with each other extremely quickly," she says. "I think in emails you give away a lot more about yourself than you would face-to-face. It got to the stage where we would email each other to say we weren't going to be there for the next ten minutes." When they eventually met, it was a bit of a letdown. "I had built him up to such an extent," says my friend, "that the reality was a letdown. But now that we're back behind our computer screens at opposite ends of the country, we're back to the way we were." If you're already in a relationship, then email is a good way to keep in touch, even if you're only apart for a day or so. Send your loved one a romantic note just to say you miss them. It might be better to save the pervy messages for when you meet, in case the boss happens to be looking when your email arrives.

Phone sex is a great way to talk your lover through how much you're missing her and what you'd like to do to her. It is guaranteed to keep the sparks flying while you're away. You'll both be looking forward to the reunion more than ever.

However, the daddy of all communication between absent lovers still remains letter writing. The fact that someone has made the effort to write you a letter in this age of rapid communications is pretty sexy in itself. If you're planning a sexy letter, think about the paper you use, whether you spray a little of your favorite scent on it to remind him of you, maybe include a photo or a small lock of hair. For tips on seductive letter writing, read the book *Dangerous Liaisons* by Choderlos de Laclos, which is entirely made up of letters. It centers on the sexy and manipulative relationship between two aristocrats and former lovers in eighteenth-century France, the Marquise Isabelle de Merteuil and Vicomte Sébastien de Valmont. The two of them play out their passionate and destructive love affair in a series of letters. It is a story about depravity, cruelty, sexual power, and deceit, but above all it shows how powerful a letter can be.

Writing is an off-putting thought for most of us who haven't lifted a pen since we were in school. Try to make writing more of a habit, and the easiest way to do this is to keep a diary. Just jot down a few lines a day to begin with. It will help you focus on your life and clarify what is important to you in each day. This helps when writing letters. Practice, practice, practice. If you're in a boring meeting at work or waiting for the doctor, then use the time to write.

If you don't want to write it, say it with a surprise. Find out how in IDEA 9, *The art of the sexy surprise.*

Try another idea...

"[Cybersex] really doesn't mean that much, it's just something that's really fun to do, that leaves no mess, no side effects, and it's the best form of contraception you'll ever find."
SIXTEEN-YEAR-OLD GIRL, quoted in *Growing up Digital* by Don Topscott

Defining idea...

161

How did it go?

Q **Nothing seems important enough to write down. What should I say?**

A *You may not think it's important but your loved one will. Remember, it's the fact that you bothered to write that is going to make them feel good. Imagine he or she is standing in front of you and say what comes into your head.*

Q **I am having a cyber romance with someone in the office. Nothing has actually happened yet but I think things are leading that way. Is this a bad idea?**

A *It depends entirely on your circumstances. If you're both single and game, then go for it. If there are other people involved, then maybe the romance should stay cyber. There is something very sexy about a cyber romance and you avoid all sorts of disappointments such as bad breath and B.O.*

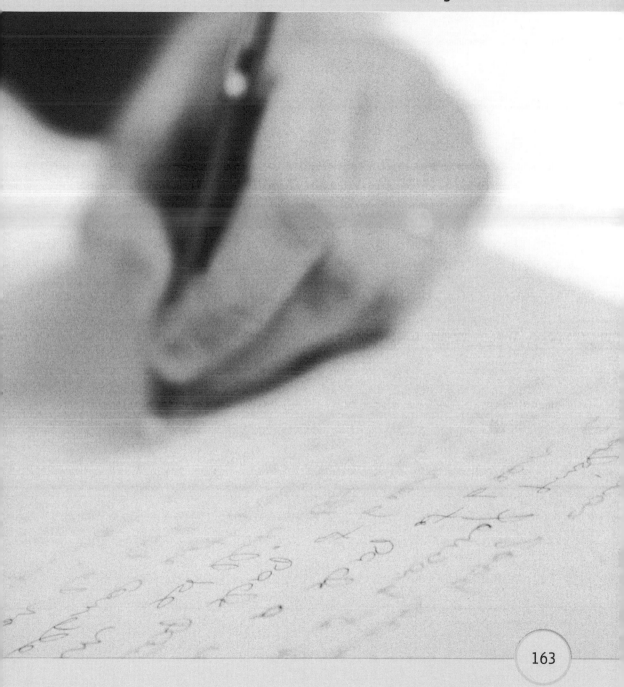

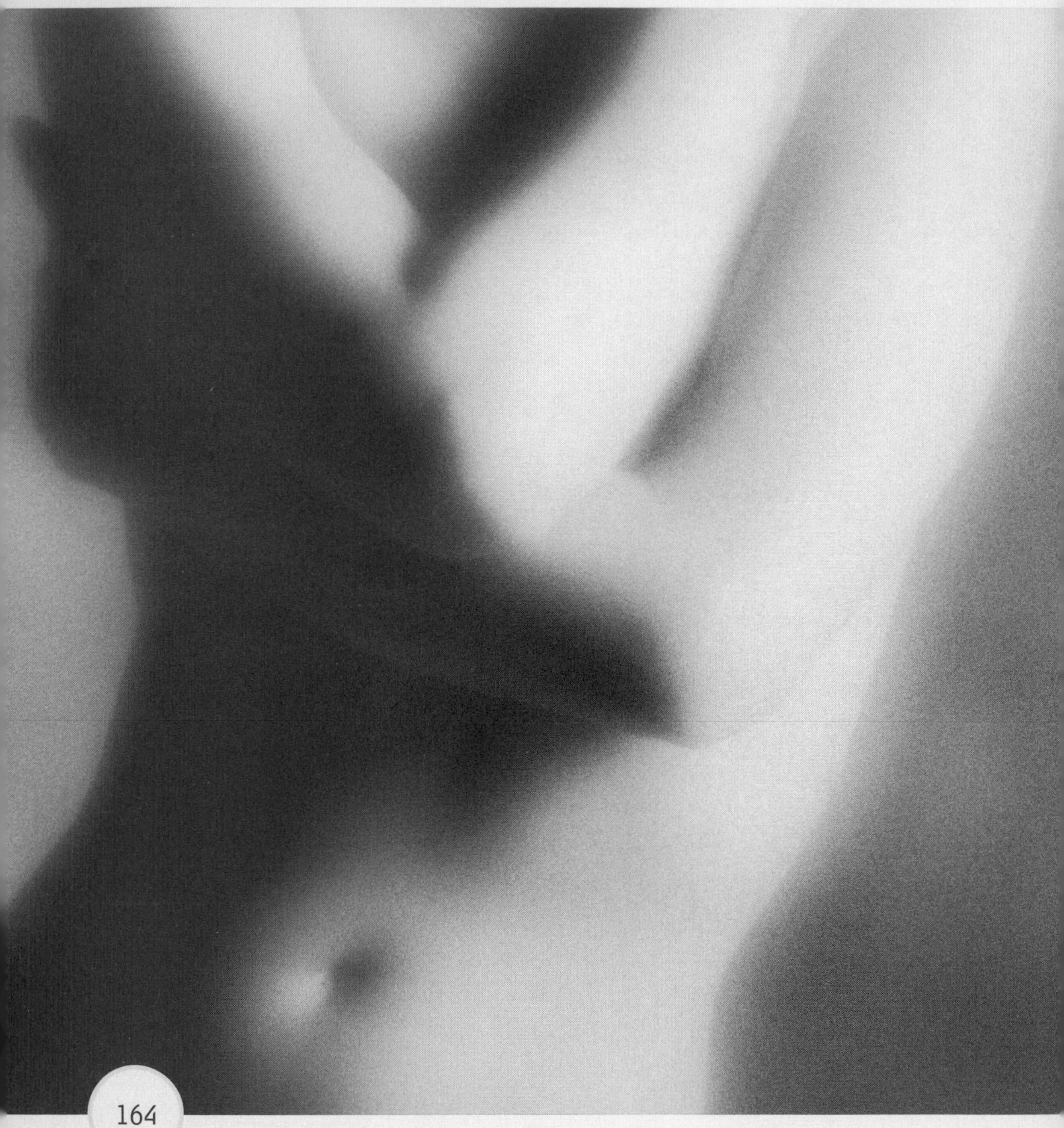

38

Beauty and the breast

All the magazines are full of images of skinny women with tiny waists and thin faces. Being a size 6 is old hat. Now we should aspire to be a size 0.

It's crazy, because one thing is for sure. The old adage that men like something they can get ahold of still stands.

If you are voluptuous, use it, play to your advantage. Wear clothes that accentuate your chest and hips, thus making your waist look thinner. Think classic movie star hourglass figure. A friend of mine fluctuates between a size 10 and 12. She is very pretty but lacked confidence, as she thought she was too fat. She spent years going on awful diets that made her feel dreadful. Still her body shape remained the same. "One day I was walking home from work, it was sunny, and I was wearing a T-shirt and long flowing skirt. My hair was loose and I was feeling quite good," she says. "A total stranger came up to me and gave me a rose. He told me he had been carrying it the whole day looking for a woman that epitomized his ideal to present it to. For the first time ever it occurred to me that I was sexy just the way I am."

Here's an idea for you...

If you are toned you will never look out of shape, no matter how voluptuous you are. You should do sit-ups, push-ups, and squats every day. Hone those beautiful curves until they are irresistibly perfect.

The fact that Marilyn Monroe was a size 14 has often been quoted. The first time I heard it, I couldn't believe it. I thought it was impossible that a sex symbol could be so, well, large. In fact, if you watch her wiggling down the platform in the film *Some Like it Hot*, you can see she really does have what you might call child-bearing hips. But there's no denying that she is one of the sexiest film stars of all time.

So the lesson is, if you've got it, flaunt it. Wear tops that accentuate your cleavage and wear bras that make the best of your breasts. If you are short, avoid horizontal stripes, as they will accentuate your size; go for vertical stripes or plain colors. Choose clothes and colors that exaggerate your femininity; long flowing dresses, pastel colors, lace (with a hint of cleavage showing, of course). If you worry about your bottom being too big, wear loose pants with side fastenings. These flatten your tummy and minimize your butt.

According to a website that celebrates the hourglass figure, the skinny ideal that we're all supposed to aspire to is only something propagated by fashion designers and marketing forces. It goes on to say that the hourglass, or pear-shaped, female form has been idolized for centuries.

Less than 3 percent of American women are the size of the models that grace the front covers of all the magazines. So 97 percent of them are "unattractive." That means an awful lot of so-called unattractive women are getting laid, falling in love, getting married, and having children every day. Go figure. It's got to be the magazines that have it wrong.

Check out IDEA 12, *The power of lovely lingerie*, for tips on how to make the most of your figure-shaping underwear.

Try another idea...

The other good news is that being slightly plump makes you look younger. Skinny women have more lines. The English poet John Dryden said: "I am resolved to grow fat and look young at forty, and then slip out of the world with the first wrinkle and the reputation of five-and-twenty." That's the poetic way of stating the unavoidable truth: As she grows older, a woman has to make a choice between her face and her butt. She can't keep both in the same condition as when she was twenty.

For that reason, Dr. Jean-Louis Sebagh, one of Europe's leading beauticians and Botox experts, recommends that women over thirty-five should not try to lose weight.

"I know that there are nights when I have power. When I put on something and walk in somewhere and if there is a man who doesn't look at me, it's because he's gay."
KATHLEEN TURNER, actress

Defining idea...

How did it go?

Q **I can't bear the size of my breasts. They are huge. I feel so embarrassed about them. What can I do to hide them?**

A *Speaking as a girl whose highlight in life was finding that at seven months' pregnant I had gone from an A cup to a D cup, I can't really muster up much sympathy for your particular problem. I suppose we all want what we haven't got, but there is no getting away from the fact that men LOVE big breasts. I don't know why, maybe it's a mommy thing, but they just do. OK, so there are things you can do to lessen your curves, bras you can buy, and certain colors and cuts of clothes that will diminish the effect, but why bother? Be proud of your chest. Carry it well, don't slouch and try to hide it. Women all over the world will be insanely jealous and men will be falling over themselves to please you.*

Q **This is all very nice, but inside every fat woman isn't there a skinny woman wanting to get out?**

A *If you're really unhappy about your size then you can do something about it. Go on a detox for a week (no dairy, no wheat, no sugar) and see how much excess weight comes off. But don't blame me if your boyfriend starts complaining.*

39

Spice up your life

Time to reinvigorate yourself with something completely different.

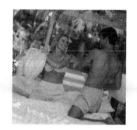

Make routine a thing of the past—and get ready to hit the Refresh button on your sex life.

Think differently from the pack. Be your own person and do your own thing. I'm not suggesting you go AWOL, but I am suggesting you use a little imagination to spice up your everyday life and increase your sexy image. Be more aware of your surroundings, look for the positive in the humdrum, and create sexy situations where you normally wouldn't.

For example, your alarm goes off at 7 a.m., you get up, shower, eat something, trudge down to the subway or the train in the pouring rain, and go to work. This happens most days. However, some days, something different will break the

Here's an idea for you...

Surprise him by offering to wash his car, wearing a short skirt and stockings and garters. The neighbors will be eternally grateful, too. Use your imagination to surprise people, including yourself!

monotony: a musician playing your favorite song, a story in the newspaper that makes you laugh, a brief glance from a fellow-commuter that sets something off in the depths of your half-asleep psyche. But to notice these things you have to be receptive and ready for them.

Try to treat each day as an adventure. It's a terrible old cliché but live each day as if it were your last. Realistically you can't do that or you would never go to work, but you get my drift. Instead of thinking, "God this is dreadful, I hate this commute" think, "I wonder what or who is waiting around the corner." Even if you're not so optimistic that anything remotely exciting awaits you on the 7:47, take something exciting with you, like a novel full of steamy sex and adventure. Try reading *Dangerous Liaisons* or *The Sexual Life of Catherine M* on the train—it will at least get the imagination going of any commuter reading over your shoulder.

In terms of your sex life and your relationship, you should adopt the same approach. "If there is a choice of what to do on the weekend, always go for the most eccentric one," says a male friend of mine who has an above-average success rate with members of the opposite sex. "I find things like ice skating or a picnic in a boat work better than a classic dinner out." Romance is something that often goes out of a relationship early on; try to keep it alive by making an effort to do things a bit differently. Think about how much it meant at the beginning that your partner had even agreed to go on a date with you. Try to recapture that feeling and hold on to it; at least for a night once in a while. Increase the sexiness and excitement of being together by doing something you don't normally do. Get on a bargain flight to a city you've never visited, spend all day in bed feeding each other strawberries, or do something you've always wanted to do but have never dared try, be it bungee-jumping or dressing up in a nurse's uniform.

Spice up your life with some massage—see IDEA 31, *Get the massage?*, for more details.

Try another idea...

If you're not in a regular relationship then try to break out of your own pattern once in a while, too. If you normally spend Saturday afternoons watching football, get off the sofa and go to a museum for once. If you're single, it's an even better idea. "Museums are a perfect prowling ground," a twenty-one-year-old male friend tells me. "They're the one place girls often go alone and you can easily strike up a conversation by asking what they think of a particular painting. And they love the fact that you're there at all, it immediately says you're the sensitive, arty type."

"Variety is the spice of life."
LATE 18TH-CENTURY PROVERB

Defining idea...

How did it go?

Q   I just can't think of anything different to do for my girlfriend's birthday. Any ideas?

A   *How about literally spicing up her life with a fabulous cooking course somewhere? There are literally hundreds advertised on the Internet, all over the world. Also, don't underestimate the value of spices; fill your pantry with ginger and spicy goodies like turmeric and coriander, then experiment with some sexy new recipes. Ginger is a great cure-all and a marvelous way to start the day. Bash a lump with the end of a knife or a pestle and pour boiling water over it—it's guaranteed to pick you up.*

Q   What about for my boyfriend's birthday?

A   *Men are easier to please, really. As long as they have food, drink, sex, and are not uncomfortable, they're pretty happy. Out of that list, sex probably comes first so for his birthday you need to come up with something that involves just that. Why not offer him one of his fantasies as a present? If that means you have to dress up in a bunny-girl outfit, then so be it. It is his birthday, after all. You could also offer to be his sex slave for a couple of hours. But make sure he returns the favor one day.*

40

Sexy dates

So, he or she has finally agreed to go out on a date with you. This is it. Make or break. You need to make sure they want to come back for more.

Although there is room for a romantic dinner or two in anyone's dating itinerary, put a bit more thought into the first date than merely making a restaurant reservation.

The most important thing to remember is that sexy dates do not necessarily mean you have sex. In fact, the sexiest dates are those that enhance desire and that tantalize you. They should leave you guessing what comes next, wanting to know more.

"I remember my first few dates with my husband," says a friend of mine. "We met during the day, went to museums, cinemas, had walks in the park, hot chocolates. Totally romantic and lovely. When we finally jumped into bed together it was wonderful, all that build-up made the whole thing more exciting."

Another friend of mine told me about a man she dated who would kiss her, passionately, at the end of each date, and leave her panting for more. "I began to wonder if something was wrong with me," she says. "I couldn't believe after the

Here's an idea for you...

Sexy dates aren't confined to those on first dates. If you've been together for a while then try something really radical like an evening class. You could do tango dancing or art lessons or learn a language together. Seeing each other master a new skill is very sexy.

kissing he didn't even ask to come upstairs. Then one day, after two weeks of tantalizing kissing, he whisked me off to Paris and seduced me the minute we got to the hotel. It was worth the wait."

Try to do something unusual to increase your sex appeal with your date. You'd be amazed at how much difference a bit of imagination and thought can make. A sexy date for a woman is one where she feels that her date has really thought about what it is she wants and planned ahead to please her. "I once got a card from a guy I had been seeing a bit of," says a friend. "In it was a coin. The card said he had booked a hotel for the weekend and I should toss the coin to decide whether or not to join him. If it was heads, I should go. I tossed the coin and of course, as it was double-headed, I had no choice! I found the whole idea so charming I couldn't resist him."

Here is a list of some sexy dates for inspiration:

1. Opera, ballet, theater, or film—not exactly original but a firm favorite with the girls. Make sure, though, it's not *Terminator 12* or something similar. Girls want a romantic film to put them in a romantic mood.

2. Dancing—mainly for the young. The romance of the high school dance is still very much remembered.

3. A walk on the beach—or by a river, or a trip on a boat somewhere. The great outdoors can be very romantic, even in the rain.

4. The city—museums, shops, cafés, bars. All the city has to offer, seen through new eyes.

If you still haven't secured the dream date then brush up on your introductory conversation by reading IDEA 5, *And what do you do?*

Try another idea...

5. A dirty weekend—the exception to the no-sex-on-the-first-date idea. Someone whisking you away for a luxurious, indulgent time is very sexy, as long as you know they're equally into you.

The top-five non-sexy dates in my opinion:

1. Anything that involves a tent.

2. Going for a beer with your buddies after work. No thanks, you go if you want to, I'll stay at home washing my hair.

3. Going to an Italian restaurant and acting all Italian and smooth.

4. Anything that involves standing on the edge of a field for hours in the freezing cold. If she wants to see you wearing shorts then take her to a beach instead.

5. Watching TV. Unless it's soft porn. And even then this should not be anywhere near the first ten dates.

On bisexuality: "It immediately doubles your chances for a date on Saturday night."
WOODY ALLEN

Defining idea...

175

How did it go?

Q What if you're taking a man out on a date?

A *Good for you. As I said in the last chapter, men are easier to please. But still try to use a bit of imagination. Maybe take him to something he is unlikely to have been to before. The theater, or maybe lingerie shopping if you think he's confident enough to handle it.*

Q I am too shy to ask anyone on a date, let alone think of different things to do. What would you suggest?

A *Then don't think of it as a date. If necessary, bring in some other friends. Suggest you all go for a walk. Don't turn it into a big deal.*

41

Sexy sex

So, the date went well. Now you've got her or him home and into bed. What happens next?

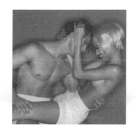

Sex is very much a participatory sport, and if your partner isn't having a good time then chances are you won't be either.

First of all, you need to get the atmosphere right. Most people find it very hard to focus on having great sex if there are disturbances. So dim the lights, take the phone off the hook, and lock the door.

Sexy sex often has as much to do with brains as positions for women. They need to be feeling right, happy, attractive, in love. Not an easy state of mind to achieve all the time. I can't stress enough the importance of creating the right mood for sex, and part of that is building suspense. Remember that seduction doesn't begin in the bedroom. Ideally, it should start the minute you open your eyes. Ways to do this include hinting at it throughout the day, by text, email, or best of all phone; showing up with some sexy new underwear for her to try on; opening a bottle of pink champagne; telling her how gorgeous she is; and creating an environment where she will feel relaxed and happy.

Here's an idea for you...

If you're a guy and want to practically guarantee that your partner enjoys herself, become an expert at oral sex. You should begin by kissing her labia in the same way you would kiss her lips, then gently caress the clitoris with your tongue, teasing her before going for the middle. At all times maintain a steady rhythm.

But even with the help of romantic music and dimmed lights, a woman won't necessarily be able to orgasm when she first goes to bed with a new partner. "I just can't have an orgasm during sex," one female friend told me. "Sometimes I feel like I'm close and then the feeling goes away again." She is probably getting in a panic and therefore not relaxing. But there are certain positions that are conducive to female orgasms that you should try if you're having trouble. For example, if the woman goes on top, then her clitoris is in direct contact with his pubic bone. If the man is on top, he can stay close to the woman, thus rubbing his pelvis or pubic bone against her and stimulating her clitoris. In other positions he can use his hand to bring her to orgasm, or she can use hers. A vibrator also comes in handy if that orgasm seems a long way away.

There are other steamy positions that can get the imagination and the body fired up. The modified missionary is a good one—basically the missionary position but with her legs over his shoulders. This increases penetration and clitoral stimulation, so it's a winner for both. But make sure that you feel supple enough for this one if you're a woman; it's uncomfortable otherwise.

Funnily enough, standing up is one of the best ways to stimulate the elusive G-spot, so try having sex against a wall or with her sitting on a kitchen stool and him standing in front of her. These positions also allow eye-to-eye contact, which makes for steamier sex. This position is also good for him as it allows him to thrust rather more energetically than some others do. Standing up or lying down from behind is another great way to get to the G-spot.

Get ethnic and exotic with Tantric sex: check out IDEA 46, *Tantalizing Tantric.*

Try another idea...

A variation on woman on top is the one where the woman turns around the other way to face the man's feet. For him it's ideal, he gets to lie back and look at her bottom. Also good for the shy woman who can't quite handle staring at someone as she writhes up and down on him. But not great for her clitoral stimulation; she'll have to do that herself. Which, incidentally, might well be the surest way of ensuring you have an orgasm with a new partner.

"A man falls in love through his eyes. A woman through her ears."
WOODROW WYATT, journalist

Defining idea...

How did it go?

Q **I'll never remember all this in bed. Is it terribly bad manners to bring a book with you?**

A *Well, it is really. But one thing you can do if you know someone well enough is to work through a chapter on positions in a sex book together. Try them out, have a laugh, and go for the ones you enjoy again and again.*

Q **Is it possible just to have normal sex and enjoy it?**

A *Of course it is, and that's probably what you'll do most of the time. This idea is for those extra steamy moments when you feel a little special.*

42

Be a cunning linguist

My father always said the only way to learn a language properly was to take a lover who speaks the language you are looking to learn.

He is Italian and speaks eight languages. My mother spoke no Italian when she met him and was fluent three weeks later. Proof that either his theory works or she is a great linguist.

People speaking several languages is very sexy. It is evidence of intelligence, sophistication (you're bound to have traveled if you speak a foreign language), and staying power (we all know learning a language is only child's play when you're a child). Americans are very bad at other languages. In Sweden, where I grew up, speaking three or four languages is not unusual.

The problem with Americans is there is not much motivation to learn another language, as everyone speaks English. But it does make you a more interesting, attractive, and sexy person, and I know firsthand that people find it fascinating when a woman can speak a foreign language well. It works for men, too. Imagine you are on your first weekend away. You have whisked her off to Paris. In the restaurant you are able to discuss the finer points of the wine list in French with the

Here's an
idea for
you...

If you buy a DVD of a foreign film, there are plenty of options. One will be the film in its original version with subtitles and another will be the film without subtitles. Try watching it with subtitles first and then without. See how much you understand. If it's impossible, go back to the subtitled version until you've got the hang of it.

sommelier. You can get around the city effortlessly and look pretty damn cool while doing so. She's going to be a lot more impressed than if you came out with a couple of phrases you last used in high school French class.

So how do we do it?

There are lots of options. The Internet is one. The BBC has very good language sites. For French, I like a woman called Laura Lawless who sends me daily lessons I never have time to read. Just key in the language you're after into a search engine and you'll get lots of options coming up. You could also enroll in a language course, but if your lessons are only twice a week then supplement them with the radio or TV programs.

In this satellite and broadband age there is no reason you can't listen to the language you want to learn in the comfort of your own home. When I first moved to France I found that listening to the radio was great for learning the language. At first I understood nearly nothing, but then I came across a news station that repeated more or less the same thing every fifteen minutes so if I hadn't caught it the first time I could listen to it again. Tune into Spanish, French, German, even Russian radio online and improve your linguistic skills.

If you find you're a natural linguist, you're probably a natural musician, too. Find out by trying out IDEA 20, *Play away.*

Try another idea...

Traveling to the country is a great way to get started. Walk around with your phrase book and try to speak to as many people as possible. The problem is that a lot of them will want to use their encounter with you as an English lesson. Set up a deal where you do half English, half the other language. Or simply join a language class. It's a great way to meet potential partners, too.

Once you have acquired a new language, of course you have to use it. Remember that your pool of potential partners has just increased dramatically. The French find French spoken with an accent very sexy. So if you've learned French, head straight for Paris. But you don't have to leave the country to show off your skills. If you've learned Italian, take your date to the opera and impress her by translating the libretto. The same goes for German, but you'd have to sit through several hours of Wagner, which might take the edge off the date.

"Life is a foreign language: All men mispronounce it."
CHRISTOPHER MORLEY, writer

Defining idea...

How did it go?

Q   It's hopeless, I'm just not a linguist. What can I do?

A   You speak at least one language, don't you? Then what's to stop you from speaking another? Just focus, immerse yourself, and you'll be amazed how much progress you can make. Be positive, like a friend of mine who started learning Russian recently. She says it is incredibly difficult but as she knew no Russian at all when she started, anything feels like a step ahead. Her aim is to meet a gorgeous Russian one day and perfect her pronunciation.

Q   So which language should I go for?

A   It helps if something about the culture intrigues you. Portuguese means you'll feel right at home in steamy Brazil. Obviously the ones that are most useful to us are those spoken in our neighboring countries. But if you want to be a bit adventurous, go for Russian (extremely sexy—think A Fish Called Wanda) or Chinese (the language of the future, apparently), and you'll certainly have a fascinating talking point when you meet someone new.

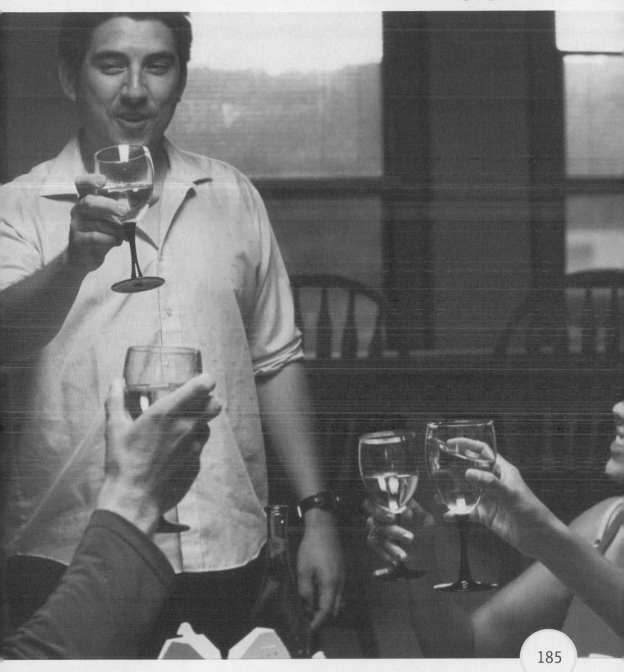

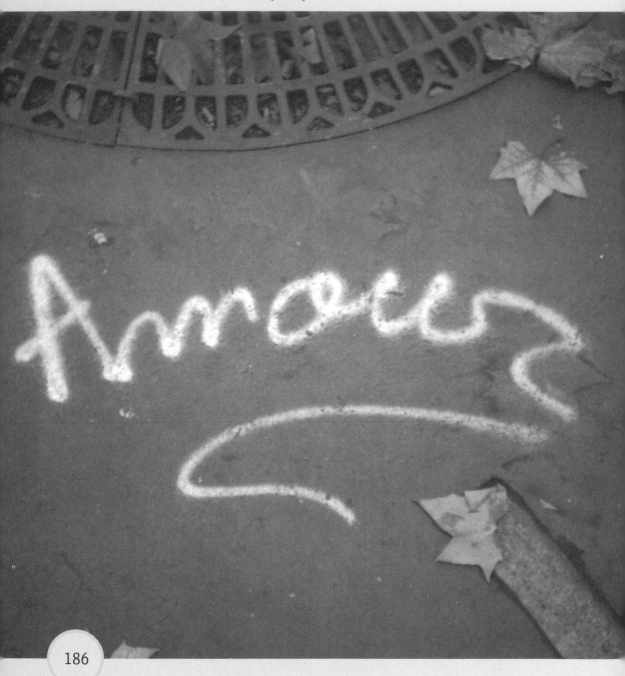

43

A certain je ne sais quoi

What is it about the French? Even their language is full of words with sexy connotations. Femme fatale, lingerie, boudoir—see what I mean?

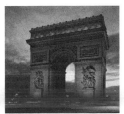

We can learn something from the French—that sometimes sexiness comes naturally and sometimes we can give it a helping hand. The effort is well worth it.

French women are very seductive. In fact, one male friend of mine went as far as to say that they are programmed to seduce. I was discussing this concept with an English friend recently. She had her Yorkshire terrier in her lap. "What do you think English women are programmed to do?" I asked. She looked at the dog and smiled. "Cuddle their dogs," she replied.

This has got to change! Girls, it's time to turn French.

Here's an idea for you...

For the French, the devil is in the detail so you must not skimp on accessories. Always buy the most expensive handbag and shoes you can. A scarf of course is de rigueur, as is the little black dress. Try to make sure you have the basics in your wardrobe and that they are good quality; the rest will follow and you will look chic and sexy effortlessly.

So how do we do this? Well, the first thing is attitude. The French are naturally confident (some would even say snotty). Where this confidence comes from, no one knows, but they do wander down the boulevards as if they own them. So you need to think French. Instill yourself with inner confidence and assurance. You are sexy, let no one tell you otherwise (especially that little self-doubting voice inside).

Frenchwomen are chic and elegant, another essential element to being sexy. So how do you suddenly acquire this innate gift? The best place to start is with your underwear. Now that you're thinking like a Frenchwoman, you will need to discard your faded cotton briefs and invest in some seriously stylish delicates. Wearing beautiful, supportive lingerie takes ten pounds off you, makes you feel marvelous, and with stylish underwear, you're unlikely to want to cover up with anything unflattering.

Makeup and hair are also essential. The fundamental mantra for most French women is "natural but not casual." So go for light lip glosses, subtle highlights, and not much eye makeup. Get your eyelashes curled and dyed by all means; it means you look great, even without mascara, first thing in the morning. Professional eyebrow shaping opens up your eyes and takes years off you.

Frenchwomen are also generally thinner than other women. Here are a few top tips from one who has lived here for five years. Despite having had three children, I am just a little over the weight I was at college. Remember, the key to eating like a Frenchwoman is moderation not deprivation.

- Order a green salad at every given opportunity

- Start with a mineral water when you arrive at a cocktail party

- Eat real chocolate

- Go for smaller portions

- Choose goats' cheese over other cheese wherever possible

- Go for olives over nuts or chips during the aperitif

- Never drink alcohol once the meal is over

Once you've mastered the attitude, master the language. Check out IDEA 42, *Be a cunning linguist*, for more on that.

Try another idea...

"Elegance is refusal."
COCO CHANEL

Defining idea...

A sense of humor and character is an essential part of the Frenchwoman package. They seem to have a rather refined, almost chic sense of humor and plenty of spirit. Don't forget that Frenchwomen come from a long line of libertines. Their culture is full of independent, sexually active women, and they take their lead from them. Read up on Colette, Anaïs Nin, and Emanuelle; they will inspire you.

Women find Frenchmen sexy, especially the way they talk. I'm not suggesting you men go around sounding like Inspector Clouseau, but think French on your next date. Take her to a local French restaurant or, better still, to one in Paris. Go to the

Deux Magots where Jean-Paul Sartre and Simone de Beauvoir drank coffee every day and philosophized.

To dress well, Frenchmen tend to dress like an English gentleman, but you could probably take some tips from them in the aftershave and personal grooming departments. It is true that they are in general better turned out than their non-French counterparts. Don't feel embarrassed about buying male beauty products; Frenchmen having been doing it for years.

How did it go?

Q   I'm about as French as a hot pot. How can I convince myself, let alone anyone else, that I'm a chic chick from Montparnasse?

A   *It's all about image and self-image. You just need to believe. Don't just read this chapter—take up the ideas. Remember: Above all, make an effort. Frenchwomen are horrified by how little time American women put into their appearance. Set aside time to pamper yourself once a week. Indulge in some lovely negligées. Nurture your femininity. Don't take it for granted.*

Q   I find it hard to define how a Frenchwoman should dress. Where can I look?

A   *You could watch some French films, there are lots of them around, except that the women rarely keep their clothes on for long. Other than that, read magazines with interviews with famous actresses like Juliette Binoche, Isabel Adjani, and Emmanuelle Béart. You could also look at what the French fashion houses are doing and consult magazines to see what the local boutique equivalent is.*

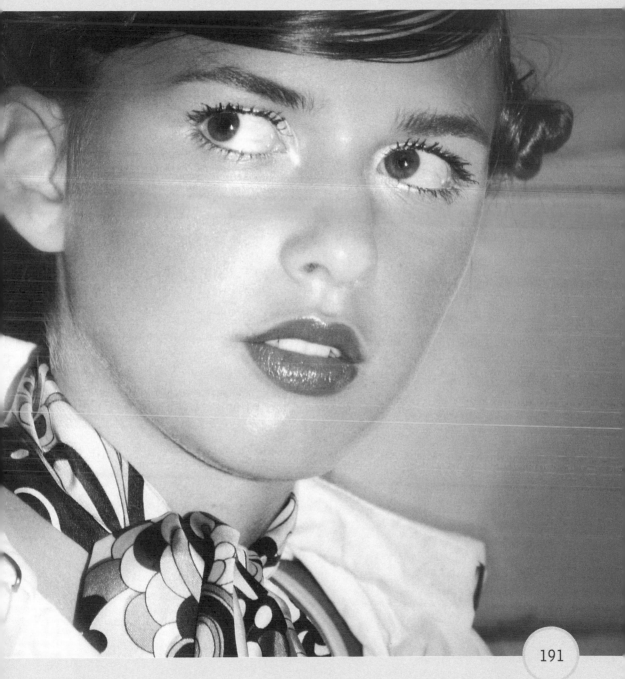

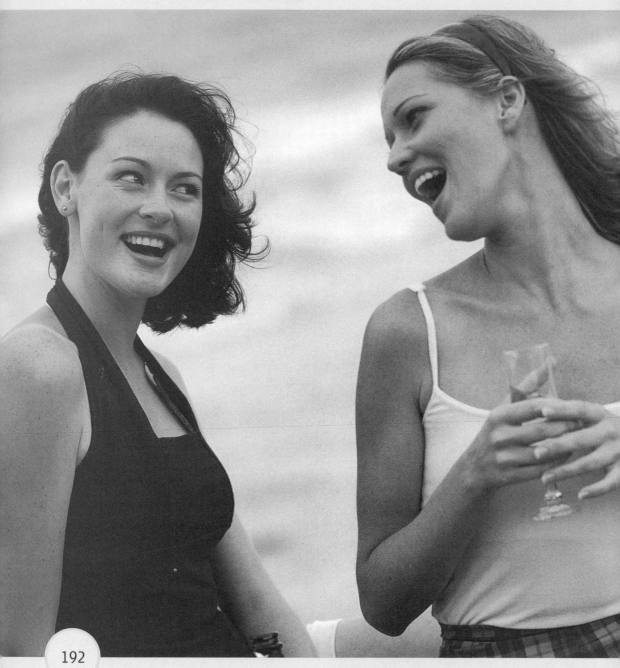

44

Make 'em laugh

You would hardly describe Woody Allen as a looker, would you? But he's still managed to get some of the most stunning and talented women around.

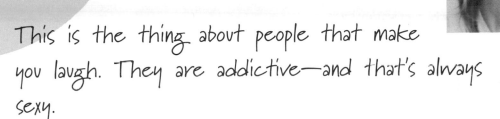

This is the thing about people that make you laugh. They are addictive—and that's always sexy.

A very attractive friend of mine was diagnosed with depression last year. This girl is almost six feet tall, a former model, wealthy, intelligent. She spent three months on the couch, popping Prozac every two minutes. The cause of this depression was a short, balding guy who you wouldn't imagine she'd give a second look to. "It was just awful," she told me a few weeks ago, now more or less back to her normal self. "He made me laugh so much that no one can replace him. Other men might be more attractive, richer, whatever, but I was totally crazy about him."

It is clinically proven that laughing is good for you. Smiling and laughing releases endorphins and hormones that make you feel good. Making people laugh is big business: There are consultancies that charge $5,000 an hour to come and tell companies how important laughing is for their staff. One survey found that people even believed that those with a sense of humor were better at their jobs.

Here's an idea for you...

Next time someone or something makes you laugh, analyze why. This will help you to understand what it is that makes someone amusing and make it easier for you to emulate them. Rent DVDs of comics who are particularly good at one-liners. Dave Allen, for example, is a great person to learn how to be funny from, as his timing is brilliant.

Dr. Ashton Trice at Baldwin College in Virginia, found that humor helped people in the workplace overcome difficult problems. So maybe my girlfriend was on to something, maybe losing her funny man was the tragedy that she perceived it to be. And if you're looking for a way to make yourself instantly sexier—get funny.

Of course, different people find different things funny. The French, for example, find it hysterical when people fall over. English humor is more sophisticated and full of irony that other nationalities find hard to understand. If you're trying to entertain people then bear in mind where they're from. Bawdy Aussie jokes are unlikely to cut it with a group of prudes from Pennsylvania. And if you're talking to foreigners, remember a lot can be lost in translation.

Being funny is about being able to think on your feet and not just coming out with the most obvious thing. Standing around telling jokes won't really make you funny (although it never does any harm to have a few up your sleeve). Rather, you need to develop your sense of humor by watching people who are funny and learning from them. Humor is notoriously tough to analyze but if you keep looking out for it then you'll start to recognize what makes other people laugh.

To be funny you need to remember a few golden rules. Timing is one of them. A comment like "nice girl, wrong planet" will only work immediately after the girl in question has come out with an inexplicable comment, not twenty minutes afterward.

If your sense of humor just isn't developing as you'd hoped, check out IDEA 42, *Be a cunning linguist*, for an alternative approach.

Try another idea...

Or think of the most eccentric reaction to a comment and go with it. You'll soon see what works and what doesn't. Humor means you laugh with someone, not at them. So it has little to do with practical jokes. Also, jokes that offend people are not humorous, so steer clear of generally offensive stuff.

Finally, if you're getting desperate, you can always rent some funny DVDs. A good laugh is good for the soul and makes everyone relax. Your date is more likely to look favorably on you if you have her in stitches all evening, even if it's courtesy of another comic genius.

"You don't appreciate a lot of stuff in school until you get older. Little things like being spanked every day by a middle-aged woman: Stuff you pay good money for in later life."
EMO PHILIPS, comedian

Defining idea...

Q **Look, I'm just not a funny person. What can I do?**

A *Laugh a lot. This gives people the impression that you are funny, even if you're not. Smile when you can't laugh. You'll find you become a magnet for women all over the world. If you want to be a real lady-killer then compile your own repertoire of humorous quotes from anthologies that you can turn into one-liners and memories of things that made you and others laugh.*

Q **How else can I become amusing?**

A *Surround yourself with funny things. Look on comedy websites, watch funny films and TV programs, hang out with amusing people. You'll soon see that some of it starts to rub off on you. Think about what makes someone funny, think about what makes you laugh, and emulate it.*

45

Be a culture vulture

Many a lover has wooed his desired into bed with words. Women are extremely impressed with a well-penned thought or beautiful quote.

If you can learn to drop the perfect quote into the conversation at the right moment, you'll have the added bonus of coming across as a great wit. Women, especially, find it hard to resist a man who knows his way around a library.

A friend of mine once went to a dinner party where she knew a well-known cad would be. Much as she desired said cad, she knew it was in her very best interest to steer clear of him. He had an appalling reputation as a scoundrel and the last thing she needed to do was to end up in bed with him. Her best friend was also at the dinner party, partly to act as a "chaperone." All was going well until the subject of *Wuthering Heights* came up. This happens to be my friend's all-time obsession. She loves anything to do with it or its author Emily Brontë. There isn't a line she doesn't know. "*Wuthering Heights* is my favorite book," piped up the cad. "I think it's the

Here's an idea for you...

A good book to invest in is the *Oxford Companion to English Literature*. It sums up plots and lives succinctly. This will put literature into context and help you to identify who wrote what and when.

most brilliant piece of literature, I just can't get over how powerful and romantic it is." My friend was lost from that moment. Her chaperone conceded defeat and wished her luck.

However much you warn them, women will not be deterred from a man who knows his Shakespeare from his Byron. And not only someone who knows it, but can appreciate it as well. Men are impressed, too, by a well-read woman. Before you complete your training as a sex god or goddess, you need to focus on your intellectual sex appeal.

Being well-read is extremely sexy. If you never studied literature at school then take some time to brush up on the basics. Take your loved one to see one of his favorite romances, but be sure you at least know the plot beforehand as you'll enjoy it more. Any reference book will give it to you, or watch the film. Franco Zeffirelli's *Romeo & Juliet* is great and the version starring Leonardo DiCaprio is so fast-moving you forget you're watching a play written over four hundred years ago.

...and another idea...

Don't get too bogged down in words. Remember the famous quote from Marilyn Monroe. "I like a man with poetry in him, but not a poet."

You should also know about the romantic poets: Keats, Shelley, and Byron. Basically, the romantic poets traveled around Italy in large shirts trying to get laid and died young. (Premature death being one of the all-time great ways to secure a romantic reputation.)

Pick up an anthology of poetry and choose the ones you like best before sharing them with your lover. And if money is no object, do this on the Spanish steps in Rome, impressing her or him with the fact that Keats died in his house on the Spanish steps. It's now a museum and well worth a visit.

Try IDEA 7, *Literal appeal*, for more tips.

Try another idea...

Reading aloud to a lover is sexy. It's intimate. It's seductive. It's caring. If you're a guy then try some Jane Austen. I never met a girl who isn't in love with Darcy in *Pride and Prejudice*. It might be a real labor of love as I have also never met a man who enjoyed Austen but she'll appreciate the effort. And if she starts to associate you with Darcy in her mind, you're in. If you want something racier then go for *Lady Chatterley's Lover* by D. H. Lawrence.

You should also be aware of the great and agonizingly depressing Russian writers, among them Pushkin and Tolstoy. Pushkin wrote a brilliant poem that has been made into an opera (the CD is wonderful) and a ballet called *Eugene Onegin*. It is all about a cad who breaks the heart of a young girl. Tolstoy wrote, among other things, *Anna Karenina* and *War and Peace*, two of the great romantic novels of all time. I have never been able to get through the latter, but the point is you don't need to read it, just know about it.

"Literature Is mostly about having sex and not much about having children. Life is the other way round."
DAVID LODGE, novelist

Defining idea...

How did it go?

Q   Oh God! Where do I start?

A   *Pick up one of those crib books, like CliffsNotes. This will teach you the basics. From there you can choose the authors you want to focus on and the works that interest you. You could also read some literary criticism, which will make you sound very learned, providing, of course, that you pretend you came up with the idea yourself.*

Q   How do I drop all this newfound knowledge casually into the conversation without sounding pretentious?

A   *Well, you don't just come up with random quotes at any old time. You need to weave them in cleverly. The point is to appear educated, sensitive, intelligent, and literary. Of course, with some home study you will actually become all of those things. You won't be faking it, and then it will come naturally.*

46

Tantalizing Tantric

The idea of Tantric sex is that instead of rushing toward an orgasm, you delay it for as long as possible in order to merge with your lover in body, mind, and spirit.

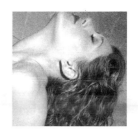

Does it sound like a lot of fiddling around for not much gain? Well, read on...

The Tantras are ancient Hindu and Buddhist scriptures that relate a dialogue between the god Shiva and his wife, Shakti. They teach us, among other things, about meditation, sex, and spiritual knowledge. In Tantric sex, the male and female energies become one, thus enhancing the whole experience for both of you.

The idea is that your sexuality is not just sex, but something that touches your whole being. The aim is to achieve a mind-blowing orgasm that propels you to heights you would otherwise not reach due to the bond between the two of you and the long buildup. It differs from western sex in that it is as much about the journey as arriving. At the very least, it will slow you down in bed, making you more aware of your reactions and those of your partner, and this alone can lead to a more fulfilling experience.

Here's an idea for you...

Take turns "spooning" each other, lying side by side. Synchronize your breathing so you are inhaling and exhaling at the same time. This has an almost magical effect in bringing you closer to each other and getting you back on each other's wavelength.

ON YOUR OWN

According to Tantric philosophy there are seven energy centers in the body, known as chakras. Each one corresponds to a color, a particular part of the body, and a certain state of mind. They are as follows:

- The base chakra, located in the pelvis. Its color is red and it is at the center of sexuality.

- The sacral chakra, just below the navel. Its color is orange and it is at the center of balance and security.

- The solar plexus chakra, at the bottom of the rib cage. Its color is yellow and it is the center of charm and self-confidence.

- The heart chakra, between the nipples. Its color is green and it is at the center of love, sharing, compassion, and joy.

- The throat chakra, on the throat. Its color is blue and it is at the center of self-knowledge and expression.

- The brow chakra, between the eyes. Its color is purple and it is at the center of imagination and perception.

- The crown chakra, just above the crown of the head. Its color is violet and it is at the center of spiritual connection and ecstasy.

To achieve the supreme orgasm, all seven chakras must be open. Focusing attention on them each in turn, on a regular basis—every day, preferably—will help you do this. Start with the base chakra, think about the color red, about the emotions and energies associated with the base chakra. Repeat this for all seven.

Check out a totally different approach in IDEA 47, _Tie me up, tie me down._

Try another idea...

TOGETHER

Tantric sex gives a whole new meaning to the word foreplay. The whole idea is to let the lust build up and then subside, thus controlling the sexual feeling to then let it explode when you have reached the required union. In practice, this usually means slowing down the man. Here's how:

1. Pull down gently on the balls. When you climax they naturally rise, so if you pull them down, they can't.

2. Visualize the sexual energy moving through each chakra rather than just the pelvis area.

3. Try the yab-yum position (yes, that really is its name), where the man kneels or sits with his legs crossed and she straddles on top with her legs wrapped around his waist and her arms around his neck. They say that if a man's spine is straight he can better control his orgasm. It also doesn't give much stimulation to the man.

"Sex is one of the nine reasons for reincarnation. The other eight are unimportant."
HENRY MILLER

Defining idea...

Even if you don't go completely for the Tantric option, why not try some of the things it suggests, like slowing your lovemaking down, appreciating and respecting each other, looking into each others' eyes. I like the exhortation to give a little bow to each other after sex. Very sweet.

How did it go?

Q **Who on earth has got time for all this?**

A *OK, so it is a little time-consuming, but remember the goal: to get closer to your partner. We should all have time for that. Treat yourself to a Tantric two days. Pick a weekend and every chance you get, dim the lights, get the soft music playing, light some incense, and start getting mystical.*

Q **My partner isn't into it. Will I benefit from doing this on my own?**

A *Yes, to a certain extent. Pick a spot in your home that is your designated meditation area. Not your bed, as this is somewhere you are going for a different style of relaxation. Light some candles if you like, strew cushions over the floor to lie on. Now lie down and breathe deeply and slowly. Repeat the chakra exercise above. Focus your mind on positive things, on things that bring you pleasure. If your attention wanders and you start worrying about things, gently bring it back to life's pleasures. Start with fifteen minutes a day and work up to half an hour. You'll be amazed how energized you feel afterward and that feeds into your sex life.*

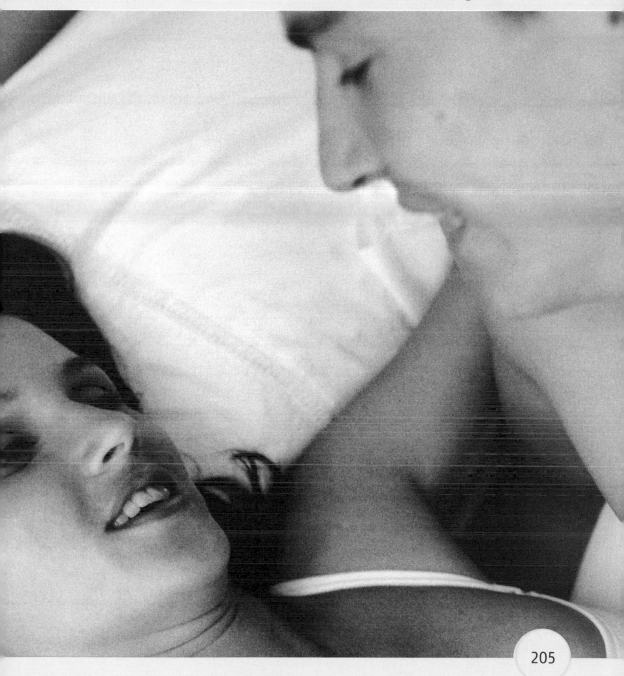

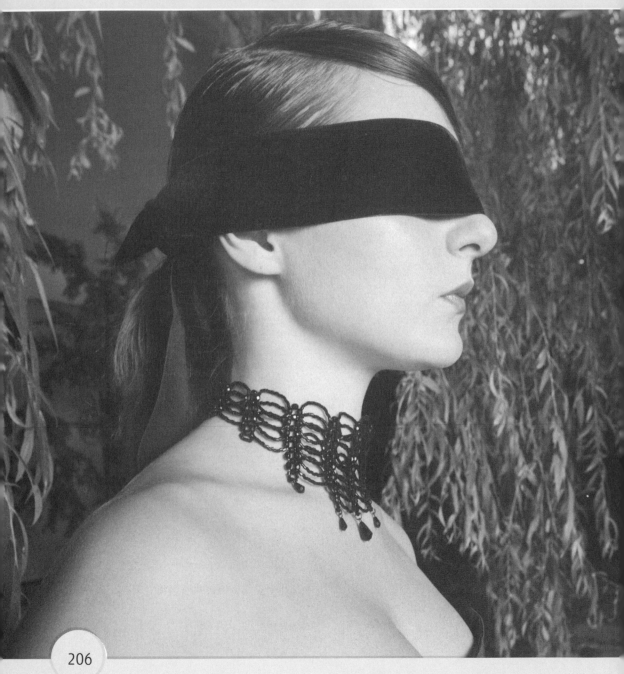

47

Tie me up, tie me down

The first time someone ties you up is a revelation. You are no longer in control and with that comes a feeling of total abandonment.

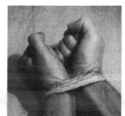

Plus, a little light bondage is always mildly pervy and that thrill of the forbidden is terrific for spicing up your sex life when you've been together for a while.

It is a fact that most men and women love to be dominated. Not all the time, but some of the time. One of the most popular female fantasies is one that involves a man forcing himself on a woman, either by tying her up or simply holding her arms down above her head. We have all read those stories of powerful men liking a good whipping by a dominatrix. What is it about bondage that turns us on?

"I just love the feeling of being totally controlled," says a girlfriend of mine. "It's like a vacation from responsibility. In life I am always the one in control, at work, at home. Sometimes it's great just to let go and be taken." Another girlfriend of mine, who forms part of the 18 percent of women in the UK who say they are "into" bondage, says it is more to do with her upbringing. "I was at a very traditional girls'

Here's an idea for you...

Create your own bondage chair by tying your partner firmly to a straight-backed chair with arms and blindfolding him or her. Or you can order your own bondage chair online.

boarding school where we were told to be coy and polite at all times," she says. "Certainly lying in bed panting for more would not have been deemed polite. This way, I am having sex supposedly against my will. What happens is beyond my control. Somewhere deep inside me a switch is turned on and I can totally relax. I just love it."

According to research, 75 percent of American men find the idea of bondage arousing (and many women do as well). I asked a male friend of mine whom I know has a penchant for it what it is that turns him on about it. "It's just nice to see a woman in that dominating role," he said. "Some of them really rise to the challenge and enjoy it. I love seeing that. And I like the fact that I'm being dominated, it turns me on to be out of control. I also enjoy the pain. Not serious agony, but the flick of the whip or the slap of a hand. There is something exquisite about the sensation, a sort of mixture of pleasure and pain you don't get from anything else."

Men tend to find women with whips in their hands very sexy. Maybe it's the fact that a woman with a whip in her hand is unlikely to be there for anything other than a serious sex session. If it's a look you haven't tried before then you might be delighted with the effect it has on your guy. Complete the image with a corset, stockings, high heels, and garters. You'll have him whimpering.

But you don't have to go the whole nine yards to get results. Even on a standard Wednesday night, tying up your lover with your tie, belt, or whatever happens to be around takes seconds and will add a delicious naughtiness to your lovemaking.

Check out IDEA 41, *Sexy sex*, for more inspiration on how to ignite your sex life.

Try another idea...

However, half the fun of bondage is that it is unusual, so you don't want to make it too mundane. Specialness is heightened if you have an armory of whips, chains, handcuffs, and silk scarves hidden away in your boudoir. If you're missing any of this essential paraphernalia then just go online and order your bondage starter kit for less than the price of a dinner for two. But be careful not to leave it lying around. My two brothers-in-law once found mine and when the rest of the family (including greatgranny) arrived for lunch they were still handcuffed to each other. Instead of the joke being on me, it had very much backfired on them, as I had gone to get some last-minute supplies and had the key with me. And that is a very important point. Never get into a lock-up situation unless you can see your get-out very firmly in front of you.

Defining idea...

"The prime ingredient that makes the power exchange work is trust. When love underlies the trust, the two partners can achieve a height of sensual satisfaction bordering on the sublime."
ALEXANDRA ADAMS, author of erotic novels

How did it go?

Q **I can't just go marching in there carrying a whip. She'll run a mile, won't she?**

A   *Probably. But you could start with a little blindfolding, then gently putting her hands above her head and seeing how she reacts. She might love it, and then little by little you can go further. The massive horsewhip on the first date is not a good idea.*

Q **How hard should you spank someone?**

A   *A very good question. Remember, some people don't get off on spanking or being spanked. So if your partner isn't up for it, don't be a pest, it will only put them off more. Instead, tempt them with some sexy literature that uses spanking to see if it whets their appetite. But remember, it may never be their thing.*

To answer your question, aim for a light spank—not enough to hurt but enough to redden the skin after a few smacks. Go gently. Spanking becomes a turn-on for the recipient after they've been spanked for a few seconds and the skin begins to tingle—if you go in too heavy, your partner won't be able to stand it long enough to get turned on. If your partner yelps and tries to hit you back, you've gone too far. This won't be good for your sex life or your relationship.

And don't forget post-spank etiquette. After the spanking, gentle stroking with a silk scarf or delicate kissing on the afflicted area is absolutely delicious.

48

Preparation, preparation, preparation

"Be prepared," they always told us in Girl Scouts. And nowhere is that motto more essential than when you're preparing for a night of passion.

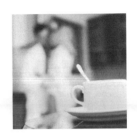

This chapter is aimed at girls. But there may be some things you guys can learn from it. Not least is how much of an effort we make for you.

Ten days until the big date. And whether you've just met or been together for years, making a bit of effort sometime before 6 p.m. on the evening of the date should make you feel better about yourself—and we know by now how important confidence is when it comes to upping the sexiness quotient.

So start your preparation early. Go on a diet. OK, so you're not going to lose ten pounds in five days, but start cutting out all nonessential foods that are likely to make you feel fat on the big night. If you have the willpower, go on a five-day detox. No wheat, no dairy, no sugar, no caffeine. Start the detox first thing in the morning with a glass of hot water, maybe with a slice of lemon in it. For breakfast have fruit if it's summer or oatmeal if it's winter. Lunches and dinners could include

Here's an idea for you... **A fun and cheaper option to a salon session is to ask one or two of your girlfriends to act as beauticians for you—obviously you'll return the favor when they need a boost to their appearance for a special occasion.**

baked potatoes with olive oil and hummus; salads with dried fruit, nuts, and legumes to give them extra substance; steamed vegetables with rice; and homemade soups. For snacks you can have oatcakes and rice cakes, with a spoonful of honey if you want. (In fact, a good substitute for tea in the afternoon is hot water and honey.) Remember to drink at least eight glasses of water every day.

Gently ease back into normal eating for the following five days. You should have clear skin, glossy hair, and a flat stomach by the end of it. On the day of your date eat small portions of fresh, healthy, non-smelly food. Avoid things that are difficult to digest, like garlic and red peppers, and fizzy drinks that can bloat you.

- *Hair*: If your hair needs remedial work—a cut or color—then book now to make sure you get an appointment at least three days before the date. If it's in good shape, at least consider a wash and blow-dry the day before or the day itself if you trust your hairdresser. There's nothing like perfectly groomed hair for making you feel terrific and it's just not possible to get the results at home.

- *Face*: A facial is a must, but should be done at least five days before the event, with a touch-up refreshing facial on the day of if you're a perfectionist (and loaded). You should also exfoliate the face, make sure your eyebrows are in order, nose hairs hidden or exterminated . . . you get the general idea. The night before the date go to bed wearing an intense moisturizing mask.

■ *Body hair*: Get rid of it two days before but not more, you don't want any stubble. A friend of mine has paid huge sums of money to have hers permanently removed by laser. "It's the best thing I ever did," she says. "No more razors, wax, or stubble."

If you're going out straight from work and haven't got time for all this then read IDEA 10, Work it!

Try another idea...

■ *Skin*: Must be smooth. Get that body brushing going, every morning. On the day of, exfoliate all over. Then moisturize.

■ *Feet*: Get rid of all that dead skin. For five days before, slather your feet in cream before you go to bed. You never know what you might be doing with them.

■ *Nails*: On no account should these be ignored. The toenails need pampering, too. See a manicurist or do them yourself in front of the TV the evening before.

■ *Underwear*: Essentially, go sexy. Most men's testosterone rises when they see red—even if women think it's a bit over the top (you can always compromise with ruby). Other men love that Calvin Klein plain white cotton look. The important thing is that the underwear is newish and matches.

"She walks in beauty, like the night of cloudless climes and starry skies."
LORD BYRON

Defining idea...

How did it go?

Q What if I don't have time to do all of this?

A *Then just do the minimum. Body brush in the morning, condition your hair, get a manicure while you're on the phone with the office, and order your sexy underwear online while checking your email. Don't arrive harassed for your date no matter how busy you are. Leave enough time to make up your face fresh before you leave the office.*

Q Will it really make that much of a difference?

A *Yes, it will to you. And as I've said all along, being sexy is all about being confident. If you think you look good, then you will.*

And that's a whole lot easier if your stomach feels flat, your hair is swinging around your head, and your skin is radiant. It also helps if you're in an outfit you've thought about in advance and chosen for its comfort as well as its looks. Don't think of this effort as being just for the man's benefit. It's far more about investing in yourself, saying "Look, I'm gorgeous, and I'm going to spend some time reminding myself how gorgeous I am." Celebrate your own sexiness regularly by making a little effort. It just so happens that other people notice, too.

49

The *cinq à sept*

The French have managed to institutionalize infidelity. They call it the *cinq à sept*, the idea being that you visit your lover on your way back home from the office in the hours between five and seven.

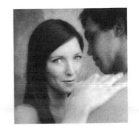

Amazingly, the people I have spoken to find nothing odd or wrong in this concept. To them the affair is perfectly normal. And if you want wanton, crazy sex, very little beats the affair.

My husband and I met at work and before we got married we had an affair. We thought no one in the office knew what we were up to, but when it finally became common knowledge one of my friends in the office said: "The only reason I thought you might not be having an affair was that you were so obvious about it." So much for our double-dealing talents. On the other hand, the French are open. "I always use the polite form of 'vous' with lovers," a male friend told me. "It's so much more sexy." And this was in front of his wife.

Here's an idea for you... **Take the five to seven literally. Meet up in a hotel room for some mad passion on your way home from work. Or get rid of the kids and go to bed *really* early.**

But I wonder if the French, for all their sophisticated acceptance of their partners' infidelities, aren't missing something. Because surely what is so sexy about affairs is that there is something totally enticing and tantalizing about the forbidden. Those moments together are so sweet because they are (a) stolen, (b) short, and (c) passionate. Combine those three factors and you have a hot situation that doesn't have a chance to burn out.

There is also the danger factor in the affair situation that makes it very exciting. Some people get addicted to this, rather like war correspondents. A male friend of mine is always having affairs with married women. "I can't stand a normal relationship now," he says. "It just seems so tedious to do normal things like the shopping, rather than just focusing on ravishing each other."

My father always says that sex is like pasta. (Well, he is Italian.) You don't want to eat the same sauce every night. He maintains that a little bit of something (or someone) different does you good and that we're too hung up on prudish fidelity. An affair can be the most exciting and wonderful thing. The sex is fantastic; intense and wanton. But of course there are huge downsides and it can all often end in tears. The problem is that one half of the unfaithful couple inevitably wants more and ends up upset and hurt because they can't just wander around the grocery store with their loved one as opposed to hanging from chandeliers with them.

It's much easier to take the wildness of the affair and translate it to your present relationship. Pretend to have an affair—with your partner. Plan to meet in a bar where no one will recognize you. Get that spark back into your relationship by treating each other like forbidden fruit; pretend to be working together or married to other people. Over drinks or dinner pretend you don't know each other, have never met. Invent another personality. Tell each other stories you've never previously shared. Surprise each other.

Role play can be a bit excruciating until you get used to it. Alcohol helps. As do props. Pretend you are having an affair with your doctor, or that your mechanic dropped in to fix a flat tire. A white coat or a whiff of gasoline will help the fantasy.

If you don't feel like having an affair, then try IDEA 39, *Spice up your life*, for other ideas.

Try another idea...

"Translations (like wives) are seldom strictly faithful if they are in the least attractive."
ROY CAMPBELL, South African author

Defining idea...

217

How did it go?

Q **I'm sure I could never be faithful to one person for the rest of my life. Are some people more predisposed to affairs than others?**

A *According to one psychological survey I read, you are more likely to have an affair if your parents weren't faithful to each other, if you have a character that craves excitement, and if you are not punctual. Some neurologists would argue that once you have had one affair, the brain pathways have been set and your mind is ready and able to do the same thing again.*

Q **Are you really recommending we all go around cheating?**

A *No, of course not. I am just pointing out why affairs are incredibly sexy and suggesting that you analyze what is sexy about them and translate what you can of it into your present relationship. Probably it boils down to: Don't take each other for granted.*

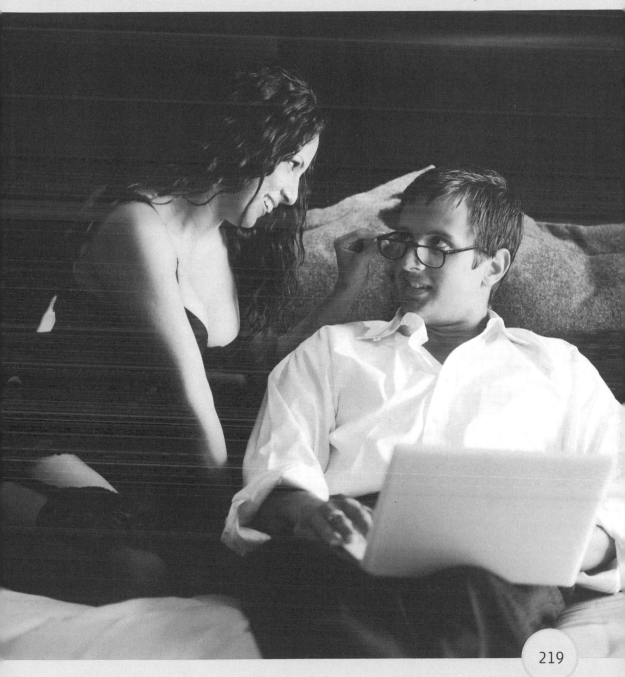

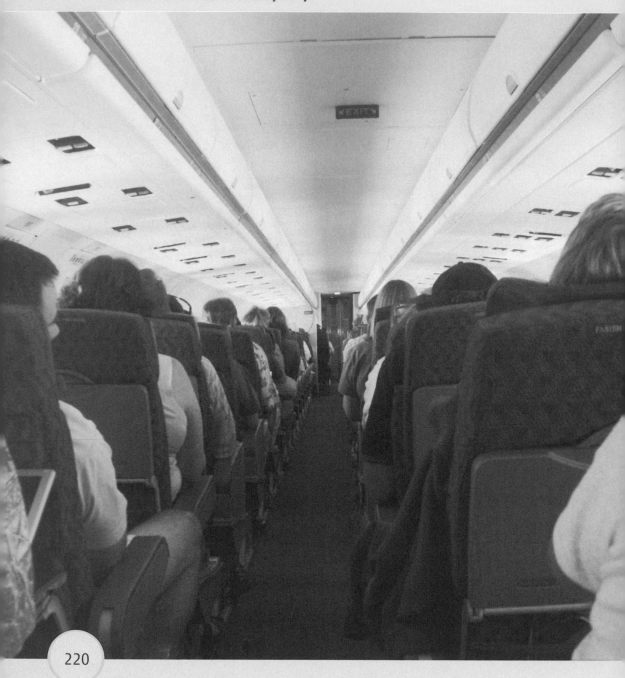

50

Sex in strange places

Beds are great, but they can get dull when you've been together for years. Even if you're not in a steady relationship, there's nothing to stop you from experimenting with sex in strange places.

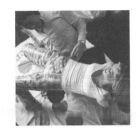

Think about it. What is the strangest place you've had sex? How was it? Exciting, weird, scary? All of the above? But the main thing is that it's memorable. Now is the time to create a few more sexy memories.

There are some obvious places to start, quite a few of them in the comfort of your own home. The shower is one: The mixture of water and sex seems to work very well. The bath is another good place. Sofas are incredibly underrated—the possibilities are endless and there's nothing like sex on a sofa to take you back to your teenage years. I have never tried swinging from the legendary chandelier but if you happen to have one, why not? Just make sure it's securely fastened.

Here's an idea for you...

Take the sex in strange places challenge—promise each other to have sex in a strange place once a week for the next two months. That's eight weird locations. Enough to have your imagination working overtime.

Objects put to a different purpose make for memorable sex. A friend once had sex on a surfboard. It wasn't actually floating on the sea at the time, but on the beach. "It was much more comfortable than you'd imagine," she said. "And certainly memorable. It was amazing how much easier it was to stay on it while having sex as opposed to actually surfing."

One French friend of mine tells me that almost everyone in France loses their virginity in a Citroen Deux Chevaux. "It's a great little car," he says. "But you have to be careful of the bar that runs across the backseat. It is hidden and can be very uncomfortable if you don't know it's there. Another good option is making love on the warm hood—*magnifique!*" Another friend of mine told me about a two-hour romp she once had in the front of a VW Golf. "It was one of the most passionate encounters of my life," she says. "But my knees were a mess for weeks afterward." Cars should not be ruled out just because you happen to be older and more sensible. A friend of mine told me she and her husband were recently driving back home from a party. They were on a deserted country road and were overcome with desire. "We stopped the car and had sex in the driver's seat," she says. "It was totally wild, partly because it was so unexpected. I'd recommend it to anyone."

The mile-high club is such a cliché I am not even going to talk about it, but just for all of you who would have written in complaining if I didn't: Yes, it is a good way to get through a long and boring flight.

I find elevators incredibly sexy places. It must be something to do with being enclosed in a small space with someone. Of course, you run the risk of being caught, which also adds to the

To go for a sexy location as well, see IDEA 28, *Location, location, location.*

Try another idea...

excitement. There is something extremely erotic about getting into an elevator with someone you have admired from afar for ages and imagining what you would do to him if that dweeb from accounting would only get out and leave the two of you alone together . . .

Having sex in public places is illegal. But if open-air romping is what really turns you on, why not try a deserted field? A girlfriend of mine once had sex with her lover in the sea off the coast of Thailand. "There were a few people in the distance, but I think they just thought we'd spotted a very interesting fish," she told me.

Sex in unexpected places is sexy partly because it is unexpected, but also because it is something new and exciting. Don't forget that to be incredibly sexy, you need to keep that edge. Dare to be different.

"I used to be Snow White . . . but I drifted."
MAE WEST

Defining idea...

223

How did it go?

Q **I can't see myself getting into all this sex-in-strange-places stuff. Can you suggest an alternative?**

A *If you don't want to go there physically, then go there mentally. Role-playing is a great way to spice things up without actually leaving home. Think of some good roles to act out, like doctors and nurses, teachers and pupils, traffic cop and illegal parker, prostitute and client, bored housewife and sexy deliveryman. The list goes on . . .*

Q **Surely this finding a strange place to have sex every week thing is a bit contrived?**

A *It's a game, and should be looked upon as just that. You have to get into the spirit of things. If you get all uptight about it then it probably will seem contrived. Relax, laugh about it, have fun with it. Get in touch with your adventurous side.*

51

Bottoms up

There are certain drinks that conjure up sexy images. There are ones that don't. A glass of pink champagne sounds a lot sexier than a whiskey sour.

Ordering a Sex on the Beach cocktail or a Long Tall Screw will only work if you are female and a mistress of irony—and even then, you'll be lucky to get away with it.

The art of drinking seductively is a difficult one. I think the French have got it right. They only ever fill up a wine or champagne glass to just below the halfway mark. This is a good idea for two reasons. First, it is much more elegant than the American habit of filling it up to the brim. Second, a lot of alcohol is not good for your sexual performance. I don't just mean in terms of men getting a hard-on, but the whole experience will be dulled by too much alcohol. As a general rule, depending on how used you are to drinking and how big you are, two glasses of wine is optimum for a woman and three for a man if you want to sparkle between the sheets. Enough to loosen your inhibitions but not enough to make you lose sight of what you're doing or desensitize you.

Here's an idea for you...

Some cocktails do work to make you feel sexy and alive. The Caipirinha (a mixture of lime, rum, and sugar) is one. Another sexy drink is the tequila slammer. Take a shot glass, pour in some tequila, put some salt on the back of your hand (or another part of someone else's body), lick it off, down the shot, and finish this off by biting hard on a lemon slice. Another variation is to fill a shot glass with tequila and lemonade, literally slamming the drink on a table hard so it fizzes, then downing it. All that licking and swallowing makes for perfect foreplay.

There is something seductive about sharing a drink with each other. The first sip loosens you up and starts the conversation flowing. Also, getting a little tipsy is a good excuse to gauge the situation if you are unsure if your intended is interested. A girlfriend of mine says that if she's not sure if her date likes her or not, she pretends to fall in his general direction. If he hangs on to her, then she knows she's got him. If not, she has another drink to drown her sorrows. I guess one could try it in an emergency.

Alcohol is marvelous for helping us to lose inhibitions, but strike a happy medium. There's nothing quite as ungainly as having passionate sex on the stairs because you just can't wait another minute, and then falling down them. That "in a heap at the bottom of the stairs with your skirt around your ears" is not a good look.

Far, far better to perfect flirting and drinking at the same time. There is the classic eyes over the rim of the glass as you take the first sip, which works for both sexes. The teasing the glass with the rim of a finger (a little contrived in my view, but expertly done by Faye Dunaway in *The Thomas Crown Affair*) can work if you're a woman and, of course, dipping one's finger in the glass and tasting it can be a winner. Anything that involves sucking fingers usually does the trick, but don't make the mistake of offering your finger to your partner to suck unless you're very sure that he or she is likely to think that's sexy.

Now that you've mastered the art of sexy drinking, see IDEA 21, *Feed your desires*, for ideas on sexy eating as well.

Try another idea...

Finally, you really can't go wrong with champagne. Take a tip from Richard Gere in *Pretty Woman*. Serve strawberries with the champagne to bring out its taste—just make sure the strawberries and the wine are top quality. This is extra good with pink champagne, by far the sexiest drink in the world. The trick with champagne is to make sure it's well chilled. You don't get that gorgeous buzz from lukewarm fizz. So get the ice bucket out in plenty of time if you plan seduction and keep the glasses in the fridge beforehand, or even in the freezer as long as you don't forget to get them out!

"Eat, drink, and be merry, for tomorrow we die."
LATE 19TH CENTURY PROVERB

Defining idea...

How did it go?

Q   **Oh God. What a nightmare! I swore I wouldn't get drunk and sleep with him and then I did. I always fail, however good my intentions are. How can I make myself stay sober?**

A   *Not easy. But in a dinner party or cocktail party situation try the following: Make the first drink when you arrive a soft one. If you have mineral water it can even look like white wine and nobody will be any the wiser. I find that once I start with wine there's no going back and I very quickly reach that point of no return when another drink becomes totally essential. If you're at a dinner party, alternate wine with water. There are actually some low alcohol wines being produced nowadays. I have heard they don't taste great, but you could try them.*

Q   **OK, I drank too much. Again. Now what?**

A   *If you're sober enough to think about it, drink as much water as you can before going to bed. When you wake up, take a dissolvable vitamin C tablet before you do anything else. Then drink some fresh orange juice, maybe with some ginger mixed in. This should perk you up. Body brush, then take a hot shower, exfoliate all over, and before you get out of the shower put it on as cold as you can get it and stand there until you've counted how many glasses of wine you drank last night. That'll teach you!*

52

Anyone for tennis?

There are certain things you just can't do as a sex god. Comic-book collecting is right up there as one of the hobbies you don't divulge to others if you want to get the guy or girl.

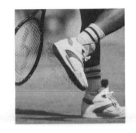

You are what you eat, the saying goes. But you are also what you do. So in your quest for sex god status, be very careful what hobbies you pick.

There are some hobbies perceived to be sexier than others. Stamp collecting is not seen as very sexy, nor is clog dancing. Sporty hobbies are generally perceived to be cooler but there are some you should avoid. Bowling, darts, and pool can all go on the non-sexy list. If you think about it, these are all sports where not much physical action is required so they can all be played by unfit people. Let's face it. The reason sportsmen are sexy is because they are in such good shape.

Here's an idea for you... **Take up life drawing. Not only will you get to see men and women pose naked but you will acquire a talent and meet new people. All of whom like naked bodies. There are life drawing classes all over the place; contact your local college for more information or look online.**

Surfing is a suitable sport for a sex god. I have always thought it looks impossible but once you get the hang of it, it's not too difficult, according to a male friend of mine. "And just wandering around the beach with a board increases your chances of getting laid by at least ten," he says.

Football is a very physical (and downright dangerous) sport. If you're relatively slim and have managed to retain your teeth, you also have the advantage on the field of being compared with a lot of larger, gummier types.

Non-sport hobbies to increase your sex god status should have a slightly intellectual bent: music, literature, art. You could take up a musical instrument or develop your knowledge and taste in music by going to concerts, the ballet, and opera. Joining a book club is a very good way for a man to get laid. They are normally made up of 99 percent women and any man who shows an interest in or an aptitude for literature will be snapped up within seconds. I am a member of a book club and we once had a man join us. He was moderately attractive and very well-read. The seven women in the group hung on his every word. In the end, I think he got so freaked out at us all staring at him and telling the others to shut up when he spoke that he never had the guts to come back. Now every month along with the question of what book we'll be reading is the question of where Christopher disappeared to and if he'll ever grace us with his presence again.

Women who knit or embroider (very Jane Austen) should do so on their own time—unless you're looking for a hipster guy who digs the crafty type. Girls could also try tennis: There's nothing men like more than a woman in a seriously short tennis skirt or dress. You could start with some one-on-one coaching—a friend of mine did this and fell in love with her tennis coach. He is ten years younger than her and is crazy for her. Her tennis hasn't gotten much better but she's always smiling.

Riding is perceived as a sexy sport for a girl, partly due to all the gear involved. It also doesn't take long before you look relatively professional, at least to the untrained eye. In that respect, it's somewhat like cycling.

Check out IDEA 11, *Fitting in fitness*, for more tips on how to stay fit and sexy.

Try another idea...

"Nobody cares if you can't dance well. Just get up and dance. Great dancers are not great because of their technique, they are great because of their passion."
MARTHA GRAHAM, dancer and choreographer

Defining idea...

How did it go?

Q   **Surely if someone doesn't love me as I am they can forget it?**

A   *Up to a point, but what we're discussing here is the initial attraction, your ability to get someone interested in you in the first place. Obviously once you're settled, it's easier to break the news that you're a secret comic book geek. But in the initial stages, image is everything and you don't want to shatter that image.*

Q   **I think geeks are quite sexy.**

A   *And you should find no shortage of pocket-protector wearers happy to indulge your fantasy. They won't believe their luck.*

Where it's at...

Index

52 Brilliant Ideas

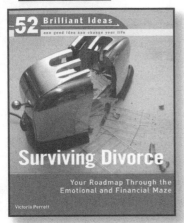

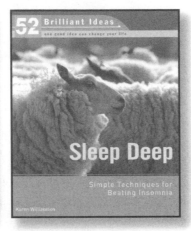

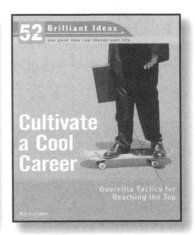

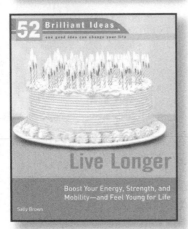

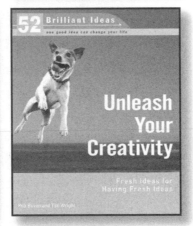

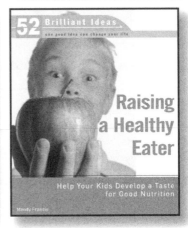

SURVIVING DIVORCE
978-0-399-53305-1

SLEEP DEEP
978-0-399-53323-5

CULTIVATE A COOL CAREER
978-0-399-53338-9

LIVE LONGER
978-0-399-53302-0

UNLEASH YOUR CREATIVITY
978-0-399-53325-9

RAISING A HEALTHY EATER
978-0-399-53339-6

PERIGEE   An imprint of Penguin Group (USA)

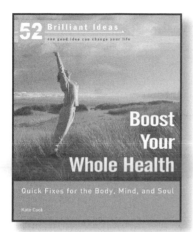
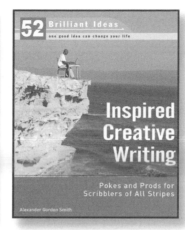
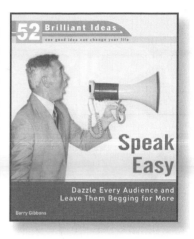
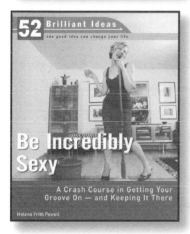
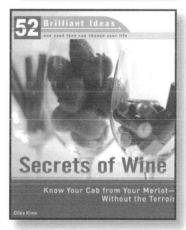
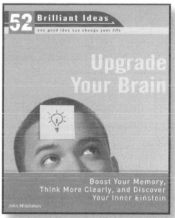